To Edna Saddler
With Best wishes
Joe F Hamburg

Your Thyroid Gland–
Fact and Fiction

SECOND EDITION

Your Thyroid Gland–
Fact and Fiction

By

JOEL I. HAMBURGER, M.D., F.A.C.P.

Northland Thyroid Laboratory
Southfield, Michigan

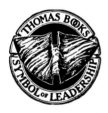

CHARLES C THOMAS • PUBLISHER
Springfield • Illinois • U.S.A.

Published and Distributed Throughout the World by

CHARLES C THOMAS • PUBLISHER

BANNERSTONE HOUSE

301-327 East Lawrence Avenue, Springfield, Illinois, U.S.A.

© *1975, by* CHARLES C THOMAS • PUBLISHER

ISBN 0-398-03375-7

Library of Congress Catalog Card Number: 74-26521

Library of Congress Cataloging in Publication Data

Hamburger, Joel I.
  Your thyroid gland.

  Includes index.
  1. Thyroid gland—Diseases. 2. Thyroid gland.
I. Title. [DNLM: 1. Thyroid gland—Popular works. WK200 H199y]
RC655.H263 1975   616.4'4   74-26521
ISBN 0-398-03375-7

Printed in the United States of America
Y-2

SPECIAL DEDICATION

To my wife Hilda, who proofread the manuscript and made important suggestions improving clarity; and to Sheldon, Paul and Daniel whose good behavior permitted Hilda to make her contribution to this work.

DEDICATION
TO THE SECOND EDITION

Since the first edition of YOUR THYROID GLAND, *Sheldon has gone off to the University of Michigan (my Alma Mater) to study engineering. Paul is completing high school. Daniel is very busy helping to keep his new brother, Aaron (born June 20, 1973) occupied so Hilda can do her proofreading.*

INTRODUCTION

THE MOTIVATION for writing this book must truthfully be acknowledged to have been *self-defense*. In my role as a consulting physician in the field of thyroid disease, seldom does a day pass without a request for suitable literature to provide a fuller understanding of thyroid problems in general, and the patient's problem in particular. As with most physicians, the time available for explanation in a busy office schedule is limited. Yet no source of information is readily available.

Furthermore, the abundance of false notions about the relationships of the thyroid gland and thyroid hormone to various symptoms seems to demand authoritative refutation. As my experience has increased over the years, the incredible enormity of this aspect of the problem has become apparent.

Hence, this book may be considered to have a twofold purpose. First, I wish to provide information, but of equal importance, I hope to dispel misinformation about the thyroid gland, its function in the body, and its diseases.

For complete understanding of the text a basic vocabulary is necessary. For this purpose a Glossary of important terms and phrases has been prepared. This will be found at the end of the book. Most thyroid patients have heard many of these words, and some even use them in their conversations with family, friends, and physicians. But it is a common observation that if one asks a person precisely what these words mean to him, frequently his understanding is cloudy, or even worse. Hence, it is recommended that the reader review the Glossary prior to reading the text, and refer to the Glossary regularly during his reading.

This book has been written for, and is dedicated to my thyroid patients, and the patients of other physicians throughout the world.

INTRODUCTION TO THE SECOND EDITION

IT IS NOW OVER FIVE YEARS since I wrote *Your Thyroid Gland—Fact and Fiction.* In general it has been well received. My own patients have found it helpful in increasing their understanding of the thyroid gland and its various diseases. Nevertheless a revision seemed in order for the following reasons:

1. The field of thyroidology is exceedingly dynamic. A number of important advances have taken place in the past few years, and these should be included in a book written to encourage informed thyroid patients.

2. In addition, certain deficiencies in the original book became apparent with time. A chapter dealing with what the patient should know about thyroid surgery seemed to be necessary. Lack of an index reduced the usefulness of the book. The problem of obesity is of such importance that it deserves the attention of a full chapter, even though this problem is not a thyroid disease. Finally, illustrations of the observable features of the various thyroid diseases were lacking.

This second edition should bring the reader up to date and correct the deficiencies of the first edition, while still keeping the book small enough to be read in one or two evenings.

CONTENTS

Your Thyroid Gland–
Fact and Fiction

Chapter 1

ANATOMY AND PHYSIOLOGY OF THE THYROID GLAND

THE THYROID GLAND is a horseshoe-shaped structure which is located at the base of the neck, astride the upper windpipe (trachea). The right and left lobes of the gland lie on either side of the trachea, and extend up the neck adjacent to the voice box (larynx). These lobes are connected by a relatively thin band of tissue called the isthmus, thus completing the horseshoe configuration. The word "thyroid" is derived from the Greek, and means shield. This is because the thyroid was thought to serve as a shield for the trachea. Figure 1 is an artist's impression of the appearance of the thyroid gland.

Thyroid tissue has a consistency approximating that of muscle tissue, hence, in most patients it can easily be examined by the fingers of an experienced physician. The total weight of the thyroid gland in normal individuals is only about one ounce; however, under abnormal conditions, it may become enlarged (goiter) and weigh several ounces, and rarely even up to a pound or more.

When very thin slices of the thyroid gland are examined under the microscope, it can be seen that the tissue is composed of numerous hollow, spherical structures (follicles) of varying sizes. The walls of these follicles are lined with the active cells of the thyroid gland. Within the follicles is a gelatinous material (colloid) containing stores of previously manufactured thyroid hormone.

The function of the thyroid gland is to produce and supply thyroid hormone in accordance with the needs of the body. Thyroid hormone is one of the basic regulators of the functions of every cell

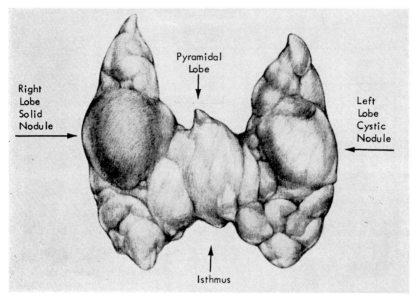

FIGURE 1. A thyroid gland (artist's conception). Note that there is a right and left lobe, a connecting isthmus and a small pyramidal lobe. Solid and cystic nodules are identified by arrows.

and every tissue within the body. Hence, it is obvious that a continuous supply of appropriate quantities of this hormone is required for good health.

To assure that thyroid hormone is made available at all times in precisely the quantities needed, despite the varying demands which arise as the result of our changing environment, the normal alterations that take place within the body throughout life, and the effects of various diseases upon body requirements for thyroid hormone, there exists a complex regulatory system of checks and balances. There is a center at the base of the brain which continuously samples the levels of thyroid hormone in the blood. This information is forwarded to the pituitary gland (located in the center of the head beneath the basal portions of the brain), which responds to a deficiency of thyroid hormone by secreting thyroid-stimulating hormone (TSH), which in turn travels to the thyroid gland and stimulates an increase in thyroidal production and secretion of thyroid hormone, thus restoring normal levels. The resultant rising concentration of thyroid hormone in the blood is then detected by the sensing device in the brain, which now alerts the pituitary to turn off its secretion of TSH. This reciprocal, or seesaw, relationship between blood thyroid hormone levels and pituitary stimulation of thyroid function, is referred to as the feedback pituitary-thyroid autoregulatory system. This may sound very complex, and difficult to understand, but if one thinks for a moment it is obvious that a very similar system is in operation every day in our homes. Consider the thermostat—furnace autoregulatory system. The thermostat detects the temperature of room air, and when it falls below a preset level, sends out a message (electrical in this case, rather than hormonal) to the furnace to put out more heat. Conversely, when the temperature rises, the thermostat detects the change and turns off the furnace. An understanding of the concept of a feedback autoregulatory system is essential to the comprehension of discussions of thyroid function tests, thyroid diseases, and the use of thyroid hormone. The reader is advised to reread the above section until he is certain that he has firmly grasped this concept.

A basic ingredient in the production of thyroid hormone is the element iodine. Iodine is present in relatively high quantities in seafood and some vegetables, and in lesser amounts in almost all fruits. Most people require only a very small quantity of iodine to fulfill the needs for thyroid hormone production. Others, whose thyroid glands are less efficient, require larger quantities of iodine. When adequate iodine supplies are unavailable, these patients will be unable to keep up with the requirement for thyroid hormone output. You will recall that according to the feedback principle of regulation of thyroid hormone production and secretion, if the level of thyroid hormone falls below requirements, a monitoring device in the brain detects the change and alerts the pituitary gland to release TSH into the circulation. This, in turn, stimulates the thyroid gland to increase its efforts to meet the demands for thyroid hormone output. Prolonged stimulation leads to enlargement of the thyroid and to goiter formation. This is why areas of natural iodine deficiency in the past were goiter belts (e.g. the Great Lakes Regions and the Alps). Millions of years ago, the glaciers removed the iodine from the soil in these areas, hence, food raised on that land was low in iodine. The significance of iodine deficiency as a cause of goiter development was first appreciated about forty years ago. This led to the introduction of iodized salt, with the subsequent marked decrease in the incidence of this type of goiter. Improved methods of food distribution have made seafood and produce from coastal areas available throughout the world. This has also contributed to a reduction in the problem of iodine deficiency. Unfortunately, there are still areas in Africa and South America where the means to prevent this type of goiter are unavailable. In some localities, one half or more of the population will have the massive goiters which have become almost unknown in more developed areas of the world. Unfortunately, even in the United States, noniodized salt is still available, and frequently is packaged in similar fashion to the iodized variety. Hence, to help protect your family from goiter, read the labels, and use iodized salt.

Chapter 2

BASIC CONCEPTS OF THYROID DISEASE— THE FOUR QUESTIONS

THE WORD "DISEASE" somehow has gained access to the list of fear words in the average person's vocabulary. I have been surprised on numerous occasions by the reactions to my use of this word in connection with medical problems. The frequent response is this, "Oh doctor, don't tell me I have a disease!" It would seem that the word "disease" means something bad, perhaps contagious, unclean, et cetera. In reality, physicians apply this word to any abnormal condition affecting the body from a cut finger to the most serious illness imaginable. If the word "disease" is used in conjunction with a thyroid problem, this is no cause for special concern or alarm. The word in this context would be completely synonymous with "illness," "condition," "problem," and "disorder."

Before discussing various thyroid diseases, it is essential for the patient to know the questions which should be asked of the physician. The questions can provide adequate understanding of the medical problem, permitting knowledgeable cooperation in a program aimed at correcting or reducing the disability of the disorder in question. We frequently hear the complaint, "My doctor doesn't tell me anything." This undoubtedly is partly the fault of the busy physician, but blame must also fall to some degree upon the patient who has not carefully thought through the information desired, and perhaps has timed the questioning inappropriately. Almost every physician can and will take the time to answer the following

four pointed questions when he has obtained adequate information
to do so.

1. *What do I have?* The patient is entitled to know, and should
   know, what is wrong. The diagnosis can almost always be
   given briefly and in simple enough terms to provide a clear
   picture of the nature of the disorder. The medical term may
   be well enough known to be employed directly, e.g. "pneu-
   monia." In most cases, simpler terms are better, e.g. "a benign
   lump in the thyroid," rather than "thyroid adenoma."

2. *What do I have to do about it?* Can it be treated with medication, or will surgery be required? This is a particularly important consideration for thyroid patients. Surgery has so
   widely been employed in the past, that almost everybody
   knows someone who has had to have thyroidectomy. Not
   only is there concern for surgery, but also for the problems
   related to the hospitalization. Arrangements are usually necessary to care for both work and household responsibilities. If
   medication alone is needed, how long will it be necessary, and
   can it be taken by mouth, or will injections be required?

3. *Will I be cured?* Patients tend to think in terms of cure or
   death. However, for many medical problems, treatment is
   aimed at controlling or arresting the progress of the disorder.
   For example, diabetes mellitus (sugar diabetes) is rarely, if
   ever, cured, but millions of people with this condition live full
   and active lives. Their disorder is under "control."

4. *What effects will the disorder have upon my future life?* This
   is a natural outgrowth of the previous question. However, the
   implications of this question are significant. Even though
   "cured," some conditions can recur. Is it necessary to alter
   one's life in any way to prevent this? Are there any complications or problems which may develop in the future? If incur-
   able, what adjustments must be made to live as well as possible
   with the disorder?

The answers to The Four Questions should prove adequate to
fulfill the needs for an understanding of the pertinent ramifications
of any illness. The application of these questions to thyroid problems is particularly helpful.

Now that we know the questions, we must review the ways in

which the thyroid gland can be abnormal.

First, there can be abnormalities of function. The function of the thyroid gland is to produce thyroid hormone, and to release (or secrete) this hormone into the blood in accordance with body needs. The thyroid hormone, secreted by the thyroid gland, is distributed widely to all the tissues and organs of the body, and is required in rather specific amounts for the proper function of these tissues and organs. Hence, a properly regulated secretion of thyroid hormone is essential to good health. If the thyroid gland produces more than the required amount of hormone, this will lead to a condition called hyperthyroidism ("hyper" means too much). On the contrary, if body needs for thyroid hormone cannot be met, the opposite condition called hypothyroidism ("hypo" means too little) develops. If function is abnormal, this problem must be corrected by methods which will either increase or reduce the blood thyroid hormone levels to normal. Abnormal thyroid gland function, both hyperthyroidism and hypothyroidism will be dealt with in later chapters.

In addition to abnormalities in the overall functional activity of the thyroid gland, one may also have disorders of its structure, i.e. size and shape. On occasion, the mass of thyroid tissue is greatly reduced, or even absent. This may result from prior surgery, radiation therapy, inflammatory disease, or rarely, as an inherited defect. More often the abnormality of thyroid gland structure is enlargement, either of the gland as a whole or a part thereof. Is is possible to have abnormal function with or without abnormal structure. When abnormalities in structure alone occur (goiter) and the proper amount of thyroid hormone secretion is maintained, the treatment required depends upon the nature of the difficulties produced by the goiter. If large enough, goiters can be cosmetic problems, and also may compress the trachea (windpipe) or the esophagus (gullet or swallowing tube), interfering with breathing or swallowing, or both. Treatment of these goiters usually requires surgery. Occasionally radiation is preferable. If the enlargement is localized to a single lump, the possibility of cancer must be considered. This will be dealt with in a later chapter.

Hence, the initial approach to the evaluation of the thyroid problem involves the determination of what, if any, functional abnormality exists, and whether or not there is goiter. Once this has been determined, the possible causes of the disorder can be considered. In the evaluation of any medical problem the physician uses three basic tools. First is the medical history. This begins with the doctor asking for the patient's principal symptom or complaint. This immediately directs the physician's thinking to the possible illnesses which may cause such a symptom, and he will ask further questions to clarify which of the possibilities seems most likely (the working diagnosis), and which of the other possibilities must be excluded (the differential diagnosis). After the principal complaint is discussed, the physician next reviews other illnesses, past or present, for these may bear more or less directly upon the reason for which the patient is seeking medical advice. Similarly, a review of symptoms relating to the function of important body organs, and a history of familial disease is often of great value. Many patients are annoyed by this routine questioning. They want something done promptly. It is important to realize that proper diagnosis is essential to proper and efficient treatment. All of the greatest physicians throughout the history of scientific medicine have agreed that the one most important technique, in fact the indispensable technique, for proper diagnosis is a careful medical history. Information obtained from the patient is frequently not subject to confirmation by the physician's own observations. Only the patient knows where it hurts, and how severe the pain is. Similarly the patient may be the only one to know how much weight he has gained or lost and how much food he eats. The term "subjective data" is applied to information of this type. In the process of diagnosis, subjective data is used primarily to obtain a working concept of the problem. The physician is much more certain of his ground if he can then confirm the working diagnosis on the basis of more concrete observations made in the course of his physical examination or by means of Xray or laboratory tests. This type of information is called "objective" data.

After the history the physical examination is performed. Even today, we are occasionally confronted by the indignant patient who cannot understand the necessity for completely disrobing for a physical examination. But to the physician, the body is like a book, and every portion is a chapter in the total story. The hair texture and distribution, the skin temperature, moisture, coloration, muscle development or wasting, size and shape of heart, liver, kidneys, and spleen, all of these and other physical findings must be checked and assessed in the light of the information uncovered by the history.

After the history and physical examination are completed, the physician usually is reasonably certain of the diagnosis. For final confirmation, and to obtain objective data on the severity of the illness, laboratory tests and Xrays may be needed. The number of laboratory tests and Xrays required varies considerably from patient to patient depending upon the complexity of the problem. Simple problems may often be treated without any testing, whereas complex problems occasionally remain unclear after the most comprehensive and exhaustive programs of medical testing. In some cases, the doctor's best diagnostic weapon is the patience to allow time for matters to clarify. It is often as difficult for the physician as for the patient to accept with equanimity the necessity of a period of indecision, when only time can solve the problem. Physicians like nothing better than clear-cut situations which yield promptly to precise, specific treatment. One of the most difficult burdens for any physician is the patient whose illness requires prolonged patience and time. In no area is this more likely than in the field of thyroid diseases. These conditions usually develop over months and years, and require equal or longer periods of time for their resolution. However, most thyroid disorders can be handled in such a way that a gratifying final result is produced.

After the history, physical examination, and laboratory studies have been completed, the diagnosis is usually established. Treatment and follow-up can then be planned, and it is possible to consider the likelihood of cure, and the future implications of the disease. As you can see, by this time, the physician has all the information needed to answer The Four Questions. Hence, the proper time to ask these questions is after his examination and tests have been completed to the point where treatment is ready to be instituted. Premature questioning of the physician is the cause of a great deal of patient dissatisfaction. Until your doctor has enough information, he cannot answer questions in a meaningful fashion. On the other hand, before treatment is started, it is important for questions to be asked and answered, for without this information, the patient is not likely to follow through with the necessary program in the most effective fashion.

Chapter 3

THYROID TESTS
AND WHAT THEY MEAN

PHYSICIANS WITH MODERN TRAINING can usually tell a great deal about the thyroid gland on the basis of a careful medical history and physical examination. For more precise determinations, thyroid tests are employed. Thyroid tests may provide information on how well the thyroid gland is performing its function, i.e. production of thyroid hormone. These tests are called thyroid function tests.

Other tests assess the structure of the thyroid gland, its size and shape, the uniformity of function throughout, or the function within certain structural abnormalities such as nodules. The physical structure of nodules may be evaluated to differentiate the cystic from solid form.

LESS RELIABLE FUNCTION TESTS
The Basal Metabolic Rate (BMR)

The basal metabolic rate (BMR) is an old test which measures the patient's oxygen consumption over a set period of time. Since the rate of oxygen consumption is related to the function of the thyroid gland, this test provides a crude measure of this function. To perform a BMR test requires occlusion of the patient's nose while he breathes through the mouth. For the test to be accurate, one must be perfectly relaxed and at ease in a resting state. For a great many patients these conditions cannot be met. The test is somewhat frightening to the average person, and few patients can travel to the physician's office, wait their turn, and still remain perfectly at ease. Because results of the BMR test have been so unre-

13

liable, it has been replaced by tests which more directly measure thyroid function.

The Achilles Reflex Test

Another test which is of relatively recent origin, and has been employed rather widely, measures the rapidity of the reflex at the ankle. The physician taps the ankle tendon with a rubber reflex hammer, and this provides a stimulus for contraction of the calf muscle. Although this is an extremely simple test, it is not accurate enough for routine use.

The Protein-Bound Iodine (PBI)

This was the first practical test which estimated the blood level of thyroid hormone. As the name indicates, the test measures iodine. Normally, most of the iodine in the blood is associated with thyroid hormone. However, a number of medicines, particularly those given for Xrays of the gallbladder and kidneys, contain large quantities of iodine. These and other iodine-containing medications can cause false elevations in the PBI. A modification of the PBI called the butanol-extractible iodine (BEI) is slightly more specific, but is still altered by Xray dyes.

The Serum Thyroxine by Chromatographic Assay

This is a further refinement of the PBI, still measures iodine content, and again has the disadvantage of interference by iodine-containing medications, particularly those given for Xray studies.

MODERN THYROID FUNCTION TESTS

The Serum Thyroxine by Displacement, T₄(D)

The lack of reliability of the older tests provided the impetus for the development of newer more sensitive and more specific methods. One of the newest and best methods for this determination was described by two Canadian physicians, Doctors Murphy and Pattee. In this test, T_4(thyroxine) is measured specifically. Recent exposures to iodine or iodine-containing medications do not alter the validity of the test data. However, the test requires careful attention to detail, and must be performed by experienced technologists to assure reliability.

The Free Thyroxine Index (FTI)

Although the T_4(D) test provides a sensitive and specific assay for the total thyroxine level in the blood, there may still be problems. The FTI is a better test which avoids these problems. Therefore the FTI is the preferred test to measure blood levels of thyroxine. For those who wish to know why, and are willing to wade through some difficult reading, the details follow. Others may just take my word for it and skip over to *T₃ by Radioimmunoassay*.

Most of the thyroxine in the blood is attached to proteins, called thyroxine-binding proteins, which serve to carry the hormone through the blood and also as a storage depot, releasing hormone to the tissues as needed. The fraction of thyroid hormone which is attached (or bound) to this carrier protein is thus not really the active form of the hormone. The active form is the tiny fraction of unbound hormone which is released from the hormone-carrier protein complex. This fraction is called the *free thyroxine*, and amounts to only about 0.1 percent of the total blood thyroxine. Usually levels of free thyroxine vary in parallel fashion with the total thyroxine level. For example, patients with excessive thyroid function (overactive or hyperthyroid) have levels of both total and free thyroxine which are higher than normal, while for patients with deficient thyroid function (underactive or hypothyroid) both levels are below normal.

However, the level of total thyroxine is dependent not only upon thyroid function, but also upon the amount of carrier protein available. If the carrier protein happens to be increased, the total thyroxine level will be elevated—even high enough to suggest the possibility of hyperthyroidism. By contrast, if the carrier proteins happen to be present in less than usual amounts, the total thyroxine level will be reduced—even low enough to suggest the possibility of hypothyroidism. Since alterations in carrier protein concentration in the blood are common, test values for the total thyroxine level (the $T_4(D)$ value) may be misleading. These alterations may result from diseases involving the liver and kidney, or in some instances on a hereditary basis. By far, the most common causes of alterations in carrier protein concentration in the blood are medications. For example, medications which contain female hormone (estrogen) will elevate carrier protein concentrations and produce high test values for the total thyroxine. Since birth control pills contain estrogens, patients taking these medications will have high total thyroxine values. Interestingly, male hormone produces the opposite effect upon both carrier protein and total thyroxine.

Even though alterations in carrier protein produced these changes in total thyroxine levels, the free (unbound) fraction of the thyroid hormone in the blood is not affected, and will still reflect the state of thyroid function accurately. It is possible to measure the free thyroxine, but this is a difficult and expensive procedure and is not done other than in research laboratories. Nevertheless, since carrier alterations are so common, the $T_4(D)$ test by itself, even though sensitive and reliable, may not give a true indication of thyroid function. To exclude the possibility of misinterpretation, it is necessary to have some information on the status of the carrier proteins, in addition to the total thyroxine concentration. This data can be obtained by a test popularly known as the T_3 test, or T_3 resin uptake test. This test is improperly named, for the name might suggest that it measures the blood level of triiodothyronine (T_3). This is not the case. The test actually measures the binding activity of the carrier proteins.

If one has values for both the $T_4(D)$ test and the T_3 test, one can calculate a value or index (the free thyroxine index) which parallels the free thyroxine concentration in the blood. Thus by a relatively simple manipulation of data from tests which are readily available in most laboratories, it is possible to avoid the errors which might result from looking only at the total blood thyroxine level. The free thyroxine index is the most important modern test of thyroid function.

The T₃ by Radioimmunoassay, T₃(RIA)

As I have indicated in Chapter 1, the thyroid produces two hormones—thyroxine (T_4) and triiodothyronine (T_3). The concentration of T_3 in the blood is much less than that for T_4, but T_3 is considerably stronger. In most instances, changes in T_4 concentration parallels those for T_3, but sometimes only one of the hormones is either deficient, or present in excess. Thus it may be necessary to check the blood levels of T_3 as well as those of T_4. The development of the radioimmunoassay technique has permitted the accurate measurement of T_3 levels, even though this hormone is present in very small amounts.

TSH by Radioimmunoassay, TSH(RIA)

If you recall, the thyroid gland function is regulated by TSH, a hormone produced by the pituitary. When thyroid levels fall in the blood (underactive thyroid—hypothyroidism) the pituitary puts out increased amounts of TSH in an attempt to stimulate increased function by the thyroid gland (in accordance with the principle of the feedback pituitary-thyroid autoregulatory system—see Chapter 1). By means of radioimmunoassay we can measure the blood level of TSH, and this is of great value in two situations:

1. Diagnosis of hypothyroidism. Whenever the thyroid gland is unable to produce enough thyroid hormone to fulfill body needs, the blood level of TSH becomes elevated.

2. Once a diagnosis of hypothyroidism has been made, and treatment with thyroid hormone tablets has been started for correction, measurement of the blood TSH level is the best test to determine whether the dose of thyroid hormone is adequate. A fall in the previously elevated TSH level to normal limits indicates that the patient is receiving all the thyroid hormone necessary.

The Radioactive Iodine (RAI) Uptake

In addition to measuring the concentration of thyroid hormone in the blood, it is often helpful to know how avidly the thyroid is concentrating iodine. It is now possible to make this determination using radioactive iodine. Radioactive iodine became available early in the 1940's as a by-product of the nuclear reactor at Oak Ridge, Tennessee. The radioactive form of the element is identical to the natural form, with the exception of an unstable structure of the nucleus that leads to the emission of radiation which can be detected by suitable instruments. Since extremely sensitive machines are employed, only minute amounts of the radioactive iodine must be given to the patient.

The test procedure is called a radioactive iodine uptake (RAI uptake), since the test determines the percentage of an administered dose of radioactive iodine which is *taken up* by the thyroid gland in a given period of time. There is more than one radioactive form (isotope) of iodine available, but most widely employed is the isotope with atomic weight of 131, conventionally referred to as ^{131}I.

Thus, the test, also may be called the ^{131}I uptake. The procedure is to give the patient a capsule containing ^{131}I. At some period later (usually 24 hours) the radioactivity emanating from the thyroid gland (which results from the ^{131}I taken up) is measured. The percentage of the total administered radioactivity can then be calculated. If the patient has hyperthyroidism (see Glossary and Chapter 5) from excessive production and release of thyroid hormone by the thyroid gland, the uptake of ^{131}I is high (usually over 35 percent in 24 hours); whereas if the patient has hypothyroidism (see Glossary and Chapter 6) the uptake of ^{131}I is low (usually less than 10 percent in 24 hours).

Confirmatory Tests for the Radioactive Iodine Uptake

There are two modifications of the RAI uptake which extend the usefulness of this test.

1. The T_3 Suppression Test. The suppression test, described by Professor Sidney Werner of Columbia University, is an extremely valuable test for the confirmation of the diagnosis of hyperthyroidism. When the RAI uptake level is between 35 and 50 percent in twenty-four hours, but the picture presented by the patient is not completely convincing for a diagnosis of hyperthyroidism, the suppression test will usually settle the question. The suppression test is based upon the principle of feedback autoregulation of thyroid function (see Glossary, *feedback autoregulatory system*). An increase in the thyroid level in the blood *normally* leads to a decrease in the function of the thyroid gland. This decrease in function will be reflected in a decrease, or suppression of the RAI uptake. However, in *hyperthyroidism*, feedback regulation is inoperative. Regardless of how high the blood levels of thyroid hormone rise, the thyroid continues to function. Therefore, the RAI uptake is not reduced (suppressed) by the administration of additional thyroid hormone. In the test itself, a rapidly acting thyroid hormone (T_3) is given for one week. If the patient has hyperthyroidism, there is no suppression of the RAI uptake. In fact, the final uptake value is often higher than the preliminary value (e.g. 35 percent before thyroid hormone is given, 40 percent after). If the preliminary uptake

is high for reasons other than hyperthyroidism, the RAI uptake after thyroid hormone will be suppressed, usually dramatically (e.g. 35 percent before thyroid hormone is given, 7 percent after).

2. The TSH Stimulation Test. A low RAI uptake may reflect disease of the thyroid gland reducing its function, medication which interferes with the uptake test, or some disorder of the pituitary which prevents release of thyroid-stimulating hormone (TSH). The TSH test will help clarify the significance of a low RAI uptake. TSH of animal origin is now commercially available for administration to patients by injection. This TSH will stimulate the thyroid gland just as would the patient's own TSH if he were producing it. If the thyroid gland is truly incapable of function, there will be a minimal increase or no increase in the RAI uptake after TSH. This is very reliable evidence that the thyroid gland is abnormal. Should the uptake increase after TSH (e.g. preliminary uptake 5 percent, uptake after TSH 20 percent), then the initial low value was either the result of interfering medication, or pituitary disease impairing secretion of TSH. To differentiate between these two final possibilities requires careful investigation of the patient's medication history, or further testing. One of the most common uses for the TSH test is in the patient who has been taking thyroid hormone for a questionable diagnosis of hypothyroidism. If a twenty-four hour RAI uptake of 10 percent or greater is produced by TSH injection, and there is no reason to suspect pituitary disease, the patient may not require thyroid hormone.

The results to be expected from thyroid function tests in hyperthyroidism (overactivity of the thyroid gland producing excessive amounts of its hormone) and hypothyroidism (underactivity of the thyroid gland producing an inadequate amount of its hormone) are summarized in Table I.

TESTS FOR THYROID STRUCTURE

The Thyroid Scan

Radioactive iodine is useful not only in the performance of the uptake test, but also in the production of the thyroid scan, or scin-

TABLE I

THE USUAL RESULTS OF THYROID FUNCTION TESTING IN
HYPERTHYROIDISM AND HYPOTHYROIDISM

	Results of Thyroid Function Tests	
Thyroid Function Test	*Hyperthyroidism*	*Hypothyroidism*
FTI	High	Low
T_3 (RIA)	High	Low
TSH (RIA)	Normal or Low	High
RAI Uptake	High	Low
T_3 Suppression Test	No Suppression	Not Done
TSH Stimulation Test	Not Done	Subnormal Response

tigram. The scan is a picture, or mapping of the distribution of radioactivity throughout the thyroid gland reproduced on paper, or sometimes on Xray film. Scans are produced by rather elaborate machines (Fig. 2) which can selectively record activity point by point. The detector moves slowly back and forth over the organ to be scanned, and the recorded activity at each point is translated on to markings on paper or Xray film until a complete scan is formed.

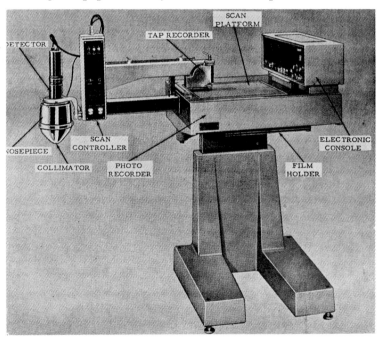

FIGURE 2. A modern scanner.*

*The Pho/Dot scanner, photograph reproduced by courtesy of Nuclear-Chicago Corporation.

Figure 3 is an example of a normal thyroid scan. Note the horseshoe shape with right and left lobes, and a connecting isthmus. It is apparent that thyroid scans provide comprehensive data on the size and shape of the gland, as well as the distribution of functioning thyroid tissue. In subsequent chapters, we will see how thyroid scanning can play a vital role in modern medical practice.

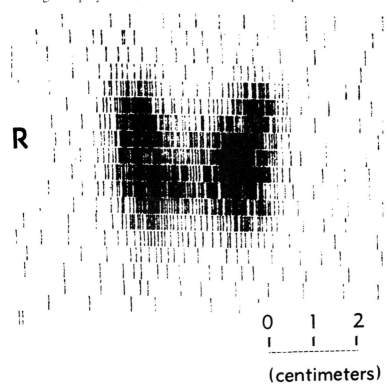

R

0   1   2

(centimeters)

V
SUPRASTERNAL
NOTCH

FIGURE 3. A normal thyroid scan. The blackened area represents the functioning thyroid tissue. The "V" over "Suprasternal Notch" indicates the location of the top of the breast bone in relation to the thyroid gland. The "R" on this and subsequent scans indicates the right side of the thyroid gland. Similarly "L" would indicate left.

Ultrasound

In the past few years there has been increasing experience with the use of diagnostic ultrasound to help in the differentiation of cystic and solid nodules of the thyroid. Most tumors of the thyroid which might have malignant potential are solid, whereas most cystic (hollow and fluid filled) nodules are benign. Therefore, this differentiation is useful. Ultrasound methods were developed on the basis of experience with sonar. You may recall that sound waves transmitted through the ocean pass unimpeded until striking a solid object, then reverberate to the transmitter. This principle is useful in determining the depth of the ocean, or in detection of submarines. If sound waves are sent through a thyroid nodule, there are continuous reverberations if the nodule is solid. These can be recorded on film as a series of a continuous spike waves (A of Fig. 4). If the nodule is cystic there will be a few spikes from the front wall of the cystic nodule, then a clear interval, and finally spikes from the back wall of the cyst (B of Fig. 4). In Chapter 7 we shall see how this information was used in a patient.

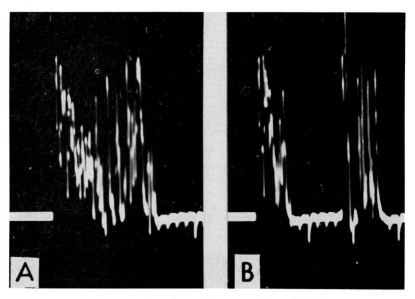

Figure 4. Ultrasound tracings for solid (A) and cystic (B) nodules. Note that the tracing for a solid nodule has continuous spikes, whereas that for a cystic nodule has a gap in which there are no spikes.

Chapter 4

GOITER

THE TERM "GOITER" seems to have many different meanings for different people. To some, it is a terribly frightening term, signifying the likelihood of death within a short period of time. Undoubtedly, these people have been conditioned to this way of thinking by an unfortunate experience in a friend or relative. For others, the term means only a minor disorder without importance. Physicians are frequently asked whether it is an "inward" or "outward" goiter. Exactly what these lay terms mean, I have never been able to ascertain. In any event, physicians apply the term "goiter" to any enlargement of the thyroid gland, whether the gland as a whole is involved, or only a portion of the gland has become enlarged. Since enlargement, per se, can be the result of almost any disease involving the thyroid gland, the determination that one has a goiter (i.e. an enlarged thyroid gland) is only the beginning of the diagnostic steps which must be taken to answer The Four Questions. As the result of these further investigations, a more specific diagnosis may be established. Clearly, the term "goiter" alone carries no implication whatsoever as to the seriousness of the disorder. A generalized, smooth, relatively symmetrical enlargement of the thyroid gland is called a "diffuse goiter." If one or more areas stand out as lumps which can easily be felt by the examining physician, the terms "nodular goiter" or "multinodular goiter" are employed.

Although there are many diseases in which goiter may be encountered, there are five mechanisms which explain the development of the vast majority of goiters. Figure 5 shows the different types of goiter which might be seen at different times in life.

COMPENSATORY GOITER

This term applies to any enlargement of the thyroid gland (goiter) which develops in an attempt to compensate for inefficient or inadequate secretion of thyroid hormone. If the thyroid gland, as the result of any disorder, becomes incapable of maintaining production and secretion of normal quantities of thyroid hormone, thy-

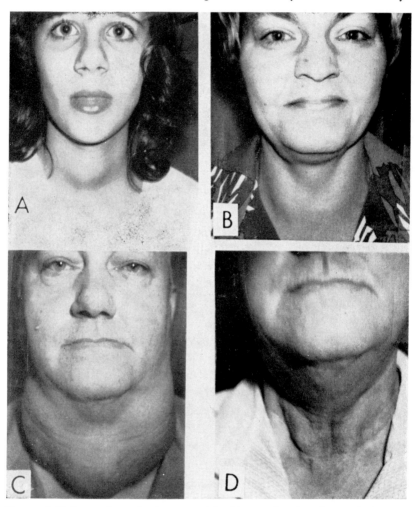

FIGURE 5. Goiter patients. A, A young girl with a small goiter. B, A middle-aged woman with an irregular larger goiter (probably Hashimoto's disease). C, An older man with a massive goiter. D, The same man after successful surgery.

roid hormone levels in the blood will fall. In accordance with the principle of the pituitary-thyroid autoregulatory feedback mechanism, there will then be an increase in pituitary TSH release in an effort to increase thyroid hormone output.

A prolonged excessive stimulation of the thyroid gland by TSH can lead to goiter formation. The causes of inadequate thyroid hormone secretion are many, but one of the most common in the world as a whole, and in years past in certain parts of the United States, is iodine deficiency. If there is inadequate dietary iodine to fulfill the needs for thyroid hormone synthesis, thyroid hormone secretion will be reduced, TSH secretion increased, and goiter will be the end result. Iodized salt has remarkably reduced the frequency of this type of goiter in many parts of the world. However, in poorly developed areas of South America and Africa, one can still visit villages in which most of the population have goiter. It is important to realize that even in the United States, where by law iodized salt must be available, many stores also carry noniodized salt. Hence, it is essential for the shopper to beware. Read the labels before purchasing salt! Compensatory goiter frequently develops following thyroid surgery. Whenever a substantial portion of the thyroid gland must be removed, the remaining tissue may be unable to maintain a normal output of thyroid hormone. Once again, there will be increased TSH stimulation of the remaining tissue with subsequent enlargement. If the original surgery had been performed for a lump or nodule, enlargement of the remaining tissue may resemble another nodule. To prevent this problem, it is best to give thyroid hormone to those who have had partial thyroidectomy for nodular goiter, if one third or more of the thyroid gland has been removed.

Another example of compensatory goiter is that which occurs in families who have a hereditary defect leading to inefficient thyroid hormone production. There are a number of steps necessary for the synthesis of thyroid hormone, and each of these steps is regulated by a special protein substance called an enzyme. Deficiencies of any of these enzymes can lead to impaired thyroid hormone synthesis. These defects may occur in isolated patients, as well as in families, and may vary in severity. If a relatively mild defect is present, the thyroid gland may be able to produce enough hormone without goiter formation under normal circumstances. However, if there is an increased demand for thyroid hormone, the thyroid gland may begin to enlarge. This is the cause of the transient goiters which are fairly commonly encountered at puberty or during pregnancy.

A number of medications may interfere with the synthesis of thyroid hormone by suppressing necessary enzymatic processes, and thus may cause goiter. Some of the more potent of these medications may be deliberately employed to slow down the production of thyroid hormone in patients with hyperthyroidism (e.g. propylthiouracil). If too much medication is used, the goiter may enlarge.

The above circumstances under which compensatory goiter may develop are not mutually exclusive. In fact, it is rather common for combinations of defects and conditions to occur, leading to mixed pictures. For example, one may see goiter development in a patient with a mild enzymatic defect, who moved to an iodine-deficient area. The enzymatic defect was not severe enough to produce goiter by itself until the extra burden of iodine deficiency was added. Figure 6 demonstrates the successful treatment of a small compensatory goiter with thyroid hormone.

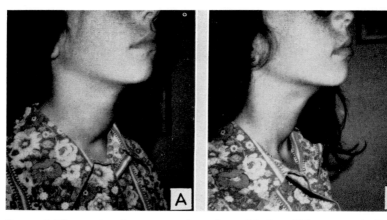

FIGURE 6. The results of treatment of a goiter with thyroid hormone. A, Before treatment. B, After treatment the goiter is much less visible.

DEGENERATIVE GOITER

Processes of degeneration may be thought of as the end result of years of "wear and tear." Throughout life, the thyroid gland is called upon to vary the production of hormone in response to the changing needs of the body. During times of increased need, the gland must increase its activity, and perhaps, even enlarge somewhat. When the need declines, the thyroid gland regresses. If this process is repeated many times, certain areas of the gland tend to remain somewhat enlarged. Small blood vessels may rupture, causing disruption of tissues, which eventually leads to scarring and even calcification of parts of the gland. Ultimately, an enlarged, irregular goiter develops with many large, nonfunctional areas. This is an important mechanism in the development of the common goiter seen in elderly people.

INFLAMMATORY GOITER

The thyroid gland is subject to infection just as any other organ in the body. Bacterial infections (acute thyroiditis) are very rare, but may become more common as the result of the increasing illegal use of drugs in this country. Attempts to inject drugs into the large veins of the neck with improperly sterilized equipment can cause bacterial infections in the thyroid gland. These are usually localized to one portion of the gland which becomes swollen, hot, and tender. The overlying skin is reddened, and the patient feels quite ill and has a high fever. Treatment requires antibiotics and surgery to drain the infectious material.

Much more common is the subacute type of thyroiditis. This is now recognized to be related to viral infections. Although subacute thyroiditis may initially develop in only a portion of the thyroid gland, usually the entire gland eventually becomes involved. Once again, the gland is tender and swollen, but to a lesser degree than is the case with acute thyroiditis. The fever, if any, is low grade. This disorder is usually treated with aspirin, but may require drugs of the cortisone type when severe. Contrary to the situation with acute thyroiditis, relapses are fairly common in patients with subacute thyroiditis. Complete recovery is the usual final outcome, but 10 to 15 percent of patients have persistent goiter or hypothyroidism, or both.

A peculiar type of inflammatory goiter has been described by a Japanese physician, Dr. Hashimoto, and thus is called Hashimoto's disease, or Hashimoto's thyroiditis. The goiter has a characteristic woody-hard consistency which seems to relate to the large amount of fibrous tissue. On microscopic examination, the tissue shows evidence of inflammation. In addition, the cells lining the follicles are larger than normal and stain a deep pink. This type of thyroiditis is being recognized much more commonly and can be seen in all age groups. The precise cause remains unknown, but current thinking is that an allergic reaction to some part of the thyroid tissue may play a role. Most of these patients have mild degrees of hypothyroidism and require thyroid horomone.

Further discussion of thyroiditis will be presented in Chapter 8.

HYPERFUNCTIONAL GOITER

The thyroid gland may, in some instances, begin to produce and secrete thyroid hormone in larger quantities than needed by the body, unchecked by the normal pituitary-thyroid feedback autoregulatory mechanism. The condition resulting from such an excess secretion of thyroid hormone is called hyperthyroidism. This disorder will be discussed in greater detail in a subsequent chapter. For now, it will suffice to say that there are three basically different types of hyperthyroidism. The most common is that described by a British physician in the 19th Century named Robert Graves, and known as Graves' disease. In this type the entire thyroid gland enlarges and becomes overactive in its output of thyroid hormone. These are the patients who may develop protrusion of the eyes (exophthalmos). Because of this finding another name for the condition is exophthalmic goiter. This illness tends to occur in women more than men by almost five to one, and although it may be seen at any age it is most common between the ages of twenty and fifty years. A second type of hyperthyroidism results from a derangement in the function of a portion of the gland. This portion, for unknown reasons, begins to function under its own control (autonomously) and secretes thyroid hormone without regard to body needs. The total secretion appears to be limited only by the mass of tissue involved and the functional capacity per unit mass. If this autonomous area becomes enlarged enough to produce more than normal quantities of thyroid hormone, hyperthyroidism will ensue. Also, since the rest of the thyroid gland remains subject to control by the pituitary-thyroid autoregulatory feedback mechanism, its function is suppresseed by the high hormonal output of the autonomous area. Hence, tissue outside the autonomous area will shrink in size, so that the enlargement is usually localized to a single mass or nodule of thyroid tissue. In the third type of hyperthyroidism, the thyroid gland is usually very large and contains many lumps or nodules. Often it is known that goiter had been present for many years, but produced no problems. When the patient reaches fifty or seventy years of age or older, the goiter then begins to produce excessive quantities of thyroid hormone and hyperthyroidism develops. Figure 7 is that of a ninety-year-old woman who had had a large nodular goiter for as long as she could remember. Ultimately the goiter produced hyperthyroidism. This type of hyperthyroidism is called toxic multinodular goiter.

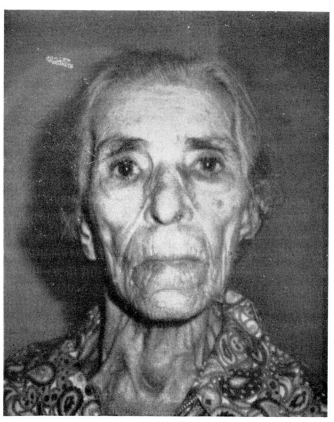

FIGURE 7. A ninety-year-old woman with long-standing multi-nodular goiter which finally caused hyperthyroidism.

NEOPLASTIC GOITER

Physcians use the term "neoplasm" (new growth) to refer to tumors, benign (adenoma) or malignant (carcinoma), which develop and grow out of control of normal body processes. Benign growths in the thyroid gland are rather common, while malignant goiter is rare. When a neoplasm is suspected, surgery is necessary. This problem will be discussed in Chapter 7.

These five basic mechanisms may occur singly or in combination, hence, the exact determination of how and why any given goiter has developed, may be exceedingly complex. Nevertheless, in most cases, it is possible to establish the principal mechanism responsible for goiter development, and thus to plan appropriate treatment.

The treatment employed for a goiter depends upon the underlying mechanism by reason of which the goiter developed. In the case of compensatory goiter, treatment with thyroid hormone is often all that is necessary. It is the deficiency in thyroid hormone which triggered the goiter formation; hence supplying this need will reverse the process. If the goiter has been present for many years, it may not regress even if thyroid hormone is taken. In these cases there is often a component of degeneration. If it is necessary to eliminate the goiter (for cosmetic purposes or because of obstruction of the trachea or esophagus), surgery may be needed.

Inflammatory goiter usually subsides when the inflammation regresses. However, the thyroid gland may be permanently damaged, and this can reduce its capacity to form thyroid hormone, leading to compensatory goiter.

The management of hyperfunctional goiter will be presented in Chapter 5.

Chapter 5

HYPERTHYROIDISM

HYPERTHYROIDISM IS A DISORDER which results from excessive quantities of thyroid hormone, either produced by the thyroid gland, or occasionally resulting from an overdose of thyroid hormone medication taken by the patient. In this section, we will discuss the picture presented by the hyperthyroid patient, and the various methods of treatment.

As previously mentioned, there are three basically different types of naturally occurring hyperthyroidism. These are illustrated in Figure 8. The more common type is that which was described by the British physician Robert J. Graves, and often called Graves' disease. Other names for this condition include exophthalmic goiter and toxic diffuse goiter, (TDG). The hyperfunction of the thyroid gland results from an abnormal overactivity of the entire gland, hence there usually is generalized thyroid enlargement. Many of these patients also have protrusion of the eyes or exophthalmos (A of Fig. 8).

Another type of hyperthyroidism is that caused by a single area of the gland which has become enlarged and nodular and which begins to secrete thyroid hormone in excess quantities on its own (autonomous function). This type of patient is shown in B of Figure 8.

The third type occurs in older patients who often have had large lumpy goiters for many years, and only late in life develop hyperthyroidism (C of Fig. 8). This type of hyperthyroidism is called toxic multinodular goiter (TMNG).

All three types of hyperthyroidism have in common the effects of the excessive secretion of thyroid hormone, but they tend to occur at somewhat different times in life, therefore the pictures are different. Table II compares and contrasts these three basic types of hyperthyroidism.

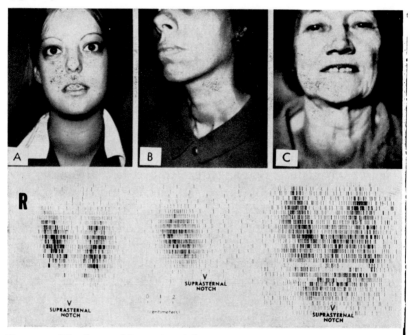

FIGURE 8. The faces of hyperthyroidism. A, A young girl with toxic diffuse goiter (TDG). B, A woman with a toxic autonomous nodule. C, An old woman with toxic multinodular goiter (TMNG).

SYMPTOMS OF HYPERTHYROIDISM

The most common symptoms of excess thyroid hormone in the body, regardless of source, are increased nervousness and irritability. Frequently associated is insomnia. However, so many people are nervous for so many other reasons, that these symptoms have very little diagnostic value. There is nothing about the nervousness of the hyperthyroid patient that is in any way different from that of the victim of anxiety or other forms of psychoneurosis.

The weight loss of the hyperthyroid patient is unusual, since it occurs in spite of a voracious appetite. In fact, the appetite is so greatly stimulated, that some patients can manage to eat enough food not only to avoid weight loss, but sometimes even to gain weight. The magnitude of the weight loss varies from a few pounds to even

TABLE II

COMPARISON OF TOXIC DIFFUSE GOITER (TDG), THE TOXIC
AUTONOMOUS NODULE, AND TOXIC MULTINODULAR
GOITER (TMNG)

	TDG	*Toxic Autonomous Nodule*	*TMNG*
1. Type of goiter	Smooth, diffuse enlargement	Solitary nodule	Large goiter with many nodules
2. Duration of goiter or nodule before hyperthyroidism develops	A few months	Many years	Many years
3. Most common age of onset	20-50 years	30-70	50-70
4. Severity of hyperthyroidism	Mild to severe	Usually mild	Mild to severe and often associated with heart complications
5. Exophthalmos	Usually	Never	Never

one hundred pounds or more, depending upon the duration and severity of the hyperthyroidism.

Because all of the tissues of the body are operating at an increased rate, the heat generated by this activity is considerable. Therefore hyperthyroid patients feel excessively warm and usually perspire profusely. Women in the menopause frequently will confuse the momentary "hot flashes" with the heat intolerance of hyperthyroidism. However, the hyperthyroid patient is warm all the time, not just intermittently.

Hyperthyroid individuals have a peculiar shakiness or tremor which is most noticeable in the hands. This can interfere with fine movements. One of our patients was a dentist and was almost incapacitated by the loss of control of his hands until his hyperthyroidism was corrected. We have also had several musicians who because of the tremor, reported difficulty in playing their instruments while hyperthyroid. The tremor may also involve the head, and less commonly, other parts of the body. A similar tremor may be seen in patients with intense anxiety and also in alcoholics.

Palpitation of the heart is characteristic. "Palpitation" means a sensation of forceful or unduly rapid heart beat. Most of us are completely unaware of the beating of the heart unless we exercise vigorously or feel for the rhythmic impulse of the heart against the chest wall. An awareness of the heart beat at rest, particularly if the rate of beating seems too rapid, is what is meant by "palpitation." This rapid heart beat, another part of the general speed-up of activity of the body processes, is characteristic of hyperthyroidism.

Loss of muscle strength can be a serious problem, particularly for the working patient. It is the larger muscles of the shoulders, hips, and thighs which are principally involved. Patients often complain that they can hardly make it up and down the stairs. This is seldom a problem unless the hyperthyroidism is severe or prolonged, or both. Figure 9 shows the loss of muscle mass which can occur in hyperthyroidism. This will improve after corrective treatment.

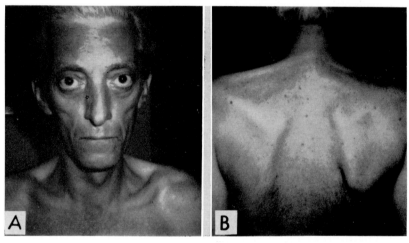

FIGURE 9. A man with hyperthyroidism which caused thinning of the chest and back muscles which control the shoulders.

The head hairs of the hyperthyroid are usually very thin, soft, and are easily extracted. Hair loss is a common problem in women. It can occur in hypothyroidism as well as in hyperthyroidism. Correction of the disorder leads to improvement. Unfortunately, most women with progressively thinning hair do not prove to have any thyroid disease.

Change in bowel habits is frequently reported. The usual patient may note an increase from one to two, or three stools daily, and the stool is softer. Occasionally, the alteration is more subtle and reflects only a change from constipation with hard movements every two to three days to normal daily movements. This point in the history may easily be overlooked unless the patient is carefully questioned.

The menstrual periods tend to decrease in volume and duration. In some patients, the reduction of flow will be to the point of just a spotting, and the exceptional patient may cease menstruating entirely. Although the concept that there is an increase in sexual drive in the hyperthyroid patient is well dispersed throughout the medical literature, in fact, the usual situation is one of decreased desire.

A group of symptoms relate to the eye problems of hyperthyroidism. There is protrusion of the eyes and retraction of the upper eyelids, which give the staring pop-eyed appearance. Furthermore, there is impairment in drainage of the tears so that the eyes water excessively. Incomplete closing of the eyelids during sleep may lead to a drying and irritation of the eyes themselves. This can cause pain, and if not attended to properly, can lead to ulceration and even loss of vision. Patients often complain of a sensation of something in the eyes, as well. Finally, sunlight and smoke cause irritation and discomfort. Figure 10 shows some characteristic eye findings seen with hyperthyroidism.

FINDINGS ON PHYSICAL EXAMINATION OF PATIENTS WITH HYPERTHYROIDISM

The physical examination reveals a nervous hyperactive patient who has difficulty sitting still, is usually perspiring excessively, and focuses upon the physician with an anxious, staring gaze. Speech is rapid fire. A goiter may be visible or may require careful examination to detect. The goiter may involve the entire gland (toxic diffuse goiter) in relatively symmetrical fashion, or less commonly, may involve one or more portions of the gland which have enlarged and present as prominent lumps or nodules (an autonomous hyperfunctioning nodule, or toxic multinodular goiter). Some diffuse goiters have multiple irregularities which seem to be small nodules. These usually occur in older patients with toxic diffuse goiter. The skin has a warm, velvety texture, and is generally moist. A pool of sweat in the navel is a common finding on examination of the recumbent patient. The hair is exceedingly fine and can be extracted with ease. Many patients are concerned about becoming bald, but the hair

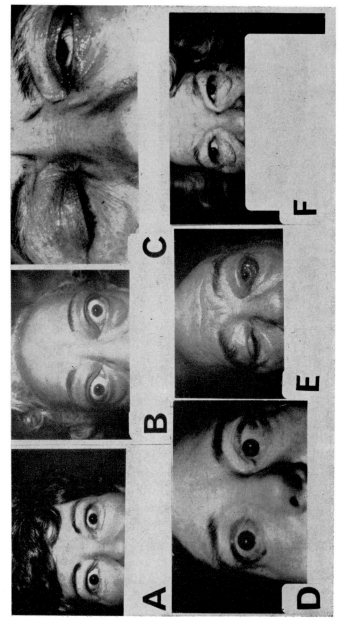

FIGURE 10. Hyperthyroid patients with involvement of the eyes. A, Retraction of both upper lids. B, Protrusion of both eyes (exophthalmos). C, Inability to close the left eye. D, Deviation of the left eye inward caused by eye muscle shortening. E, Inflammation and protrusion of the membrane which covers the eyeball, and swelling of the eyelids—especially the left. F, Swelling under the eyes in a patient who became hypothyroid after thyroid surgery.

almost always grows back after successful treatment. Tapping a muscle tendon with a reflex hammer produces an accelerated response. The outstretched hands are tremulous. The blood pressure is usually slightly elevated and the pulse rate is generally over one hundred beats per minute.

Certain less common changes occur which may be observed on examination. The fingernails may partially separate from the fingertips. This is called onycholysis (A and B of Fig. 11). The tips of the fingers may swell. This is called acropachy or clubbing (C of Fig. 11). There may be thickening and discoloration of the skin over the lower leg. This is called pretibial myxedema (D of Fig. 11). The only one of these findings to improve after the hyperthyroidism has been corrected is the onycholysis (B of Fig. 11).

LABORATORY TESTING IN HYPERTHYROIDISM

The results of laboratory testing in hyperthyroidism have been reviewed in Chapter 3. To summarize, the FTI, T_3(RIA) and RAI uptake values are elevated. The scan will show the size, shape, and distribution of functional activity in the goiter, and will help in the differentiation of toxic diffuse goiter, the toxic autonomous nodule and toxic multinodular goiter (see Fig. 8). Figure 12 shows the scans of a toxic diffuse goiter (A) before and (B) after successful treatment with radioactive iodine. Note that the general shape of the functioning tissue remains the same after treatment; only the size of the gland is reduced. Figure 13 shows the scans of a toxic autonomous nodular goiter before and after successful treatment with radioactive iodine. Note that before treatment all function was confined to the nodule (A of Fig. 13), whereas after treatment the nodule no longer functions, but the rest of the gland resumes function (B of Fig. 13). Figure 14 shows an elderly patient with a large toxic multinodular goiter. Note the appearance of the scan before and after treatment (C and E of Fig. 14). Evidence of an irregular heart beat can be seen on the pretreatment electrocardiogram (D of Fig. 14). The improvement after treatment is obvious (F of Fig. 14).

TREATMENT OF HYPERTHYROIDISM

The treatment of hyperthyroidism is a complex subject. There are three important aspects to the treatment: (1) control of the excess production and secretion of thyroid hormone, (2) elimination of

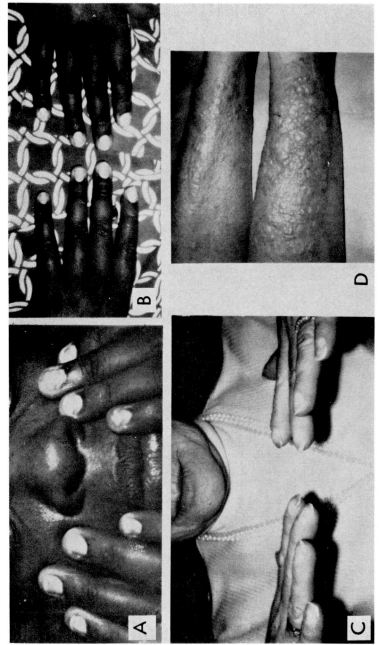

FIGURE 11. Onycholysis. A, Note the appearance of the ends of the nails in this hyperthyroid woman. B, After treatment the nails are normal. C, Acropachy. Note the swelling of the ends of the fingers. D, Pretibial myxedema. Note the changes in the skin over the legs.

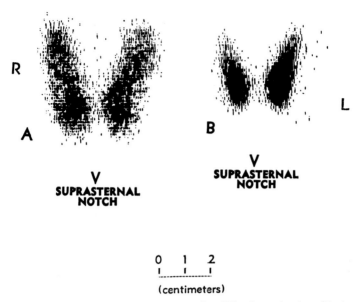

R

L

A

B

V
SUPRASTERNAL
NOTCH

V
SUPRASTERNAL
NOTCH

0   1   2
I___I___I
(centimeters)

FIGURE 12. Scans showing the appearance of a diffusely toxic thyroid gland before (A) and after (B) treatment with radioactive iodine.

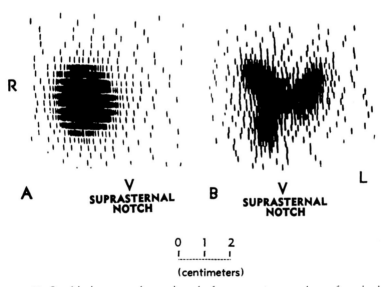

R

L

A

B

V
SUPRASTERNAL
NOTCH

V
SUPRASTERNAL
NOTCH

0   1   2
I___I___I
(centimeters)

FIGURE 13. In this instance the patient had an autonomous hyperfunctioning nodule (A) which had suppressed the function of the normal thyroid tissue. After radioactive iodine therapy (B) the nodule is no longer functioning, hence the normal thyroid tissue is reactivated.

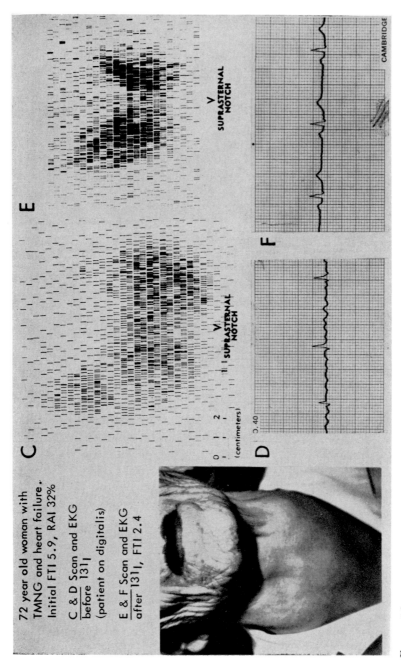

72 year old woman with TMNG and heart failure. Initial FTI 5.9, RAI 32%

C & D Scan and EKG
before 131I
(patient on digitalis)

E & F Scan and EKG
after 131I, FTI 2.4

Figure 14.

goiter, and (3) control of the effects of hyperthyroidism on any body organs or tissues, whose functions may be impaired by the large quantities of thyroid hormone circulating in the blood stream. Since the third aspect of the problem is often rather technical and involves consideration of many organs and systems, it is beyond the scope of this book. Our remarks will be confined to a discussion of methods to reduce the thyroid hyperfunction and eliminate the goiter. There are three types of treatment available for this purpose.

Surgery

The oldest, of course, is surgery. If one removes a portion of the thyroid gland, the functional capacity is thereby reduced. Superficially the treatment sounds simple, actually it is not. First medication must be given to reduce thyroid gland function and to restore the patient to good health prior to surgery. Surgery for hyperthyroidism was a very dangerous procedure with a high mortality rate before pretreatment with antithyroid drugs and iodine drops was employed. Depending upon the severity of the hyperthyroidism, adequate preparation of the hyperthyroid patient for surgery may take from four to twelve weeks. At surgery, precisely the correct amount of thyroid tissue must be removed, neither too much nor too little. It is impossible consistently to achieve perfection in a technical procedure of this type. Consequently there are some patients who are not cured by the surgery, and others who have too much of the gland removed, so that the remaining tissue cannot produce enough thyroid hormone to prevent the development of hypothyroidism. The more thyroid tissue removed, the less the chance of a recurrence of the hyperthyroidism after surgery, but the greater the likelihood of hypothyroidism. Since most surgeons are primarily concerned with curing the hyperthyroidism, the tendency is to leave only a small amount of thyroid tissue. Hence a considerable proportion of patients treated surgically ultimately require thyroid hormone replacement medication. Fortunately, this treatment is simple and inexpensive.

More of a problem is injury to the parathyroid glands, four tiny glands which are located adjacent to the thyroid gland. They are difficult to identify and easily removed, or their blood supply may be damaged during thyroid surgery. Parathyroid injury results in derangement of the regulation of blood calcium levels, which may cause convulsions, and even cataract formation. Although this problem is treatable, the treatment is difficult and requires relatively frequent visits to the physician, and laboratory tests. Another surgical complication is damage to the nerves controlling the voice. Mild voice changes are common; therefore patients for whom any limitation in the voice would be undesirable, e.g. singers or actors, should avoid surgery for hyperthyroidism. Finally, surgery carries with it a small but inevitable risk of mortality. With modern preparation and in the hands of an experienced surgeon, the mortality of thyroidectomy should be no more than one or two per thousand operative procedures. Nevertheless, this consideration cannot entirely be disregarded. Because of the complications of surgery and the requirement for hospitalization, physicians have sought safer and better methods of treating hyperthyroidism.

Antithyroid Drugs

In the 1940's medication was developed which can be given in pill form to suppress the function of the thyroid gland. There are a number of these "antithyroid" drugs, but those used most widely in the United States are propylthiouracil (PTU) and methimazole (Tapazole®). For the first time, it was possible to treat hyperthyroidism without surgery. The antithyroid drugs actually are not curative. They merely suppress the hyperthyroid process, and if the suppression is maintained long enough (about 1-2 years) the disease may cease to be active. However, it was not long before it became clear that this treatment was unsuccessful for many patients. Although the hyperthyroidism could be controlled in almost every instance, in half or more of the patients the disorder promptly recurred when the medication was discontinued. Treatment failures were more likely the older the patient, the larger the goiter, and the more severe the hyperthyroidism. Some patients with particularly severe hyperthyroidism could not be controlled in a reasonable period of time, even with extremely large doses of the medication. Furthermore, there were reactions to the drugs. These included skin rash and reduction in the while cells of the blood, thus reducing resistance to infection. Fortunately these complications clear spontaneously when the medications are stopped.

When antithyroid drugs are employed, the usual plan is to treat the patient for one to two years, then withdraw the medication and determine whether or not a cure has been produced. The antithyroid drugs are now used primarily for children or young adults with small goiters and mild hyperthyroidism. In my experience with patients older than twenty years, less than one in five will have a good result from antithyroid drug treatment. Antithyroid drugs may be given to control hyperthyroidism in children until they reach an age at which we might be willing to give radioactive iodine therapy. Antithyroid drugs also are used to prepare hyperthyroid patients for thyroidectomy, and are used to control hyperthyroidism in pregnant patients. Since the antithyroid drugs will cross the placenta to the fetus, they must be given in the smallest possible dose to pregnant patients. After delivery the antithyroid drugs can be stopped and radioactive iodine given if the patient has a recurrence of hyperthyroidism.

Radioactive Iodine

The newest treatment for hyperthyroidism, and the treatment which is being employed for more and more hyperthyroid patients every year, is the so-called "atomic cocktail" or radioactive iodine. Radioactive iodine (^{131}I) initially became available shortly after World War II, as a by-product of the nuclear reactor at Oak Ridge, Tennessee. The first physicians to use this medicine were quite unaware of what the effects would be, both long term and short term. The first question, of course, was whether the treatment would work. Could hyperthyroidism be cured by radioactive iodine? It was known that the thyroid would concentrate iodine, and therefore, radioactive iodine. It was also known that treatment with an x-ray beam could control hyperthyroidism in some patients. However, x-ray treatments deliver radiation to all adjacent tissues in the neck, whereas the principal radiation given off by radioactive iodine travels less than one eighth of an inch in tissue and would not affect tissues outside the thyroid gland proper to any degree. Therefore, on theoretical grounds, radioactive iodine seemed to be an ideal medication with which to deliver radiation to the thyroid gland to control hyperthyroidism. Very quickly it became evident that patients with hyperthyroidism could be restored to normal thyroid function and

the goiter eliminated, usually with only a single treatment of radioactive iodine.

SAFETY OF RADIOACTIVE IODINE THERAPY

Next came the question of safety. Although it was soon clear that
there were no immediate reactions, neither pain nor discomfort
nor swelling (in fact, the lack of any reaction made it difficult to
convince the patient that this small drink of "water" would really
cure him), what the long-term complications might be were initially
in doubt. There were three principal problems which had to be
considered. Since the thyroid gland received a relatively large dose
of local radiation, the possibility of the development of thyroid cancer was suggested. One can produce thyroid cancer in rats with
small doses of radioactivity, provided the rats are specifically bred
to be tumor producers, are kept on a low-iodine diet, are given
certain medications to promote tumor growth, and are given just
the right amount of radioactive iodine, neither too much nor too
little. If it could happen in rats, even very special rats, could it
happen in humans? Furthermore, tumors in other tissues have been
known to develop after x-ray treatments, and tumors of the human
thyroid gland have occurred after x-ray treatment to the thymus
of the newborn. Similarly, thyroid tumors have been detected following x-ray treatment for acne and other conditions in young
adults. Since these tumors tend to become detectable about ten years
after the radiation therapy, the likelihood of radioactive iodine treatment causing thyroid cancer could not be assessed until enough
patients had been treated and followed for a long period of time.
Since radioactive iodine has now been used for over thirty years,
it is possible to say that the initial concern for the production of
thyroid cancer was groundless. In fact, there have been fewer thyroid cancers in patients who received treatment with radioactive
iodine than would have been expected in a similar number of people
at random. It has been shown that this treatment impairs the ability
of thyroid cells to reproduce. This may in part explain the failure
of even the expected number of thyroid tumors to develop.

Since radioactive iodine passes through the blood circulation on
the way to the thyroid gland, the possibility of some effects on the
blood has been raised. It is known that victims of radiation from

atomic bomb explosions may develop leukemia. The onset of leukemia after radiation exposure takes place within a few years. Hence, it is relatively easy to evaluate the risk of this potential complication. Recently, a very large study on this point was carried out with the cooperation of twenty-six medical centers. Thirty-six thousand patients were tested to compare the incidence of leukemia in hyperthyroid patients treated with radioactive iodine with those treated surgically. When the final returns were in, in spite of the large number of patients studied, there were only forty-four cases of leukemia in all. Furthermore, there was no difference in the incidence for the two forms of treatment. Since the frequency of leukemia in patients treated with surgery was no different from that in patients treated with radioactive iodine, it would not seem likely that the treatment has any bearing upon the development of leukemia. Additional information on this point is obtained from studies on the many patients who have now been treated for thyroid cancer, using approximately one hundred times as much radioactive iodine as is employed for hyperthyroidism. Even in these patients leukemia is a rare complication.

As the radioactive iodine passes through the blood, there inevitably is some radiation to the reproductive organs. In the beginning, there was no way to judge the amount of radiation, so that the possible affects on either fertility or heredity could be assessed. Over the years these techniques have been developed, and it is now known that the radiation to the sex organs produced by the usual dose of radioactive iodine in the treatment of hyperthyroidism is approximately equivalent to that received in standard x-ray tests of the gastrointestinal tract. These levels are well within acceptable limits. Many women have become pregnant after radioactive iodine therapy, and there are no reports of fetal abnormalities. In fact, a sizeable group of young girls with thyroid cancer, treated with doses of radioactive iodine greatly in excess of those used for hyperthyroidism, have also been followed through marriage, pregnancy, and delivery, and all have normal babies.

On the basis of the above experience it is now clear that the initial concern for cancer, leukemia, infertility, and hereditary effects from radioactive iodine therapy of hyperthyroidism, seems to have been greatly overemphasized. Because of the excellent safety record with this treatment, every year more and more patients are being given the benefit of this peaceful use of atomic energy. A recent survey indicated that about forty thousand hyperthyroid patients are now being treated with radioactive iodine annually in the United States alone. Although physicians were initially reluctant to treat patients less than forty to fifty years of age, these arbitrary age limits have come tumbling down to a point where radioactive iodine is now an accepted method of treatment for all adults, and in some centers it is even being given to hyperthyroid children.

The average hyperthyroid patient can be treated with radioactive iodine in the doctor's office or clinic. Hospitalization is necessary only for the very severely ill patient or the patient with cardiac complications. Even these patients can sometimes be treated as out-patients if they are prepared for the treatment with antithyroid drugs. For ease of administration the medication is now given in a capsule rather than the earlier liquid form. There is no pain or other reaction. After the patient takes radioactive iodine, he usually experiences beginning improvement in three to six weeks. By about two months, there is substantial improvement, and within three months, most of the patients are well.

There are two methods of treatment with radioactive iodine. The standard method is to administer a single dose large enough to assure a cure in almost all patients. This approach produces the simplest, quickest and most economical elimination of the hyperthyroidism. It has the drawback that most patients will require thyroid hormone tablets permanently after the treatment is over to prevent the development of hypothyroidism. However, this is generally considered a reasonable price to pay for a prompt, simple, safe and economical solution to a major illness.

Some physicians have advised the use of lower doses of radioactive iodine in an attempt to avoid the necessity for treatment with thyroid hormone pills later. My own experience with about 600 patients given smaller doses of radioactive iodine has not been satisfactory. Many still required thyroid hormone pills, others had prolongation of the hyperthyroidism for even more than one year, and still others who seemed to do well initially, relapsed and developed a recurrence of hyperthyroidism one or more years after the treatment. Because the use of smaller doses of radioactive iodine produces uncertain results, this method is considered less satisfactory than the standard full dose approach.

Iodine Solution

Highly concentrated solutions of iodine have been employed in the treatment of hyperthyroidism for many years. Lugol's solution is the usual form. Primarily this medication is given as part of the preparation of hyperthyroid patients for surgery. The suppressant effects of Lugol's solution on the hyperactive thyroid usually lasts no more than a few weeks, hence it is not generally employed for long-term treatment. However, an occasional patient with very mild hyperthyroidism, and minimal thyroid enlargement may be treated successfully with Lugol's solution alone. This treatment has the advantages of safety, simplicity, and economy. Unfortunately, these advantages are available only to very few hyperthyroid patients. In some cases, after treatment with radioactive iodine, hyperthyroidism, although much improved is still slightly active. For these patients, Lugol's solution also may be given for six to twelve months with success.

Beta-Blocking Drugs

An important recent advance in the treatment of hyperthyroidism has been the development of drugs which can block some of the effects of high levels of thyroid hormone. Some of these effects may be the result of an influence upon otherwise normal hormones (particularly adrenalin) produced by the central part of the adrenal glands. When blood levels of thyroid hormone are increased, the body responds as if there were an excess of adrenalin; for example the heart races and the hands become shaky. The beta-blocking drugs, of which propranolol (Inderal®) is the one most generally employed, can relieve these symptoms while permanent treatment is planned. Propranolol also can be used to relieve the temporary hyperthyroid symptoms which may occur in patients with subacute thyroiditis (see Chapter 9).

SPECIAL CONSIDERATIONS WITH HYPERTHYROIDISM

Neonatal Hyperthyroidism

Newborn infants of mothers who have, or have had hyperthyroidism (of the Graves' disease type) may have a temporary form of hyperthyroidism which is thought to result from a transfer of an abnormal thyroid stimulating substance from the mother to the infant. The infant is able to eliminate this substance in a few weeks, hence neonatal hyperthyroidism is only a temporary condition. The infant will have goiter, rapid heartbeat, restlessness and may lose weight. The addition of iodine solution to the formula is all that is usually needed to control the condition.

Childhood Hyperthyroidism

Hyperthyroidism may occur at any age. It is most common in the twenty to fifty-year-old population. However, teenagers may have it, and less often it may be seen in younger children. The youngest child I have seen with hyperthyroidism was only five years old. The risks of surgery in children are somewhat greater than adults, hence most physicians prefer medical treatment. The usual plan is to administer antithyroid drugs for one to two years. If the hyperthyroidism ceases, the antithyroid drugs may be stopped. Otherwise the medication may be continued until the patient is old enough to give radioactive iodine. Although some authorities recommend radioactive iodine for children, most prefer to avoid this treatment until the patient is fully grown. The possibility that radioactive iodine in growing children may predispose to a subsequent development of thyroid cancer has been suggested. So far those who treat children have not observed this problem, but more experience is needed before radioactive iodine can be considered routine treatment for hyperthyroidism in children.

Hyperthyroidism in Pregnant Patients

This is a rare combination of conditions. Hyperthyroid patients seldom become pregnant since their fertility is reduced. When it does occur the physician must be concerned not only with the mother, but also with the fetus. Radioactive iodine is not given to pregnant patients, for it might affect the fetal thyroid, especially if the pregnancy is past the tenth week. Surgery may increase the risk of miscarriage. Hence the usual treatment is antithyroid drugs. It is important to use the smallest possible dose since these medications do cross over to the fetus. The mother should be checked every three to four weeks during the pregnancy. This is necessary for hyperthyroidism tends to improve as pregnancy advances, and therefore it is necessary to decrease the dose of the antithyroid drug. With careful management excellent results can be obtained, both in terms of control of the mother's hyperthyroidism, and in terms of the baby's welfare.

Hyperthyroidism and Heart Disease

Almost all patients with hyperthyroidism have rapid heart rate, and thus complain of palpitation. This stimulation of the heart may be little more than an unpleasant complaint for young healthy patients; but elderly patients, particularly those with a heart weakened by age or previous heart disease may have more serious trouble, including heart failure and abnormal heart rhythms. These patients require careful management of the heart problem as well as treatment of hyperthyroidism. The usual plan for thyroid treatment is to control hyperthyroidism with antithyroid drugs, and then administer radioactive iodine for permanent control.

Thyroid Crisis or Storm

This is a very severe and fortunately rare form of hyperthyroidism. The heart rate (pulse rate) may reach extreme levels, even more than 150 beats per minute. There is fever, and often nausea, vomiting and diarrhea. These patients are obviously desperately ill. Thyroid crisis may be precipitated by surgery or infection. Treatment includes cortisone, large doses of antithyroid drugs, iodine intravenously and the beta-blocking drug, propranolol. With prompt and precise management, dramatic improvement may be seen within twenty-four hours.

Summary—Treatment of Hyperthyroidism

In summary, there are three effective methods for the treatment of hyperthyroidism: surgery, antithyroid drugs, and radioactive iodine. As time goes by, surgery is employed less and less for this purpose. The more common modern indications for surgery are obstructing goiters which do not respond to radioactive iodine, or those for which there is concern for thyroid malignancy. Antithyroid drugs, as a curative treatment, are used primarily for children and young adults with mild hyperthyroidism and small goiters. For most of the remaining patients radioactive iodine is the treatment of choice.

Treatment of Exophthalmos

The exophthalmos which accompanies hyperthyroidism in some patients is an independent problem, and the development of this complication may or may not parallel the course of the hyperthyroidism itself. Nevertheless, control of the hyperthyroidism is an essential first step in the management of the eye problems. If the eyes improve, nothing more need be done. However, in the exceptional patient, as the hyperthyroidism is brought under control the eyes begin to worsen progressively. Management of these patients is extremely difficult and may ultimately require surgery to enlarge the bony cavity in which the globes reside. In most instances the end result is satisfactory, but patience is required, for it may take many months of treatment before the eye problems are brought under control.

Treatment of Pretibial Myxedema

Another peculiar and poorly understood complication of hyperthyroidism is a change in the skin over the front part of the leg, referred to as pretibial myxedema. The skin of this area may become thickened, raised, and somewhat inflamed. Why this should develop in association with hyperthyroidism is unclear. It is a rare complication occurring in probably less than one percent of all hyperthyroid patients. A new and effective treatment has been devised employing Saran Wrap® after the application of a cream containing a cortisone-like drug. This may be done nightly for several weeks until the skin problem improves. There is a definite tendency for recurrence, however, and repeated treatment is often necessary.

Hypothyroidism After Radioactive Iodine Therapy

The one complication of radioactive iodine therapy for hyperthyroidism is hypothyroidism. The precise dose of radioative iodine needed to cure any given patient of hyperthyroidism is difficult to determine even with considerable experience. The greater the experience the better the results, but it seems clear that any treatment for hyperthyroidism which eliminates a significant proportion of the thyroid tissue will ultimately give rise to a high incidence of hypothyroidism. The remaining tissue simply is unable to maintain the necessary thyroid hormone production for the rest of the patient's life. It is important to recognize that hypothyroidism may develop many years after treatment with radioactive iodine, or for that matter, after thyroidectomy as well. Some patients will ultimately become hypothyroid even when only treated with antithyroid drugs, a method which does not destroy thyroid tissue. Perhaps there is somewhat of a tendency for the thyroid gland which has been overworked for any period of time to fail prematurely. Therefore all patients who have been treated for hyperthyroidism, even though thyroid function has been restored to normal, should be seen by their physicians at least once yearly on a permanent basis. Hypothyroidism may develop very gradually and insidiously and may not be recognized by the patient. However, modern testing can often predict the onset of hypothyroidism before it is far advanced. Hypothyroidism is much simpler to correct when still mild, than after it has become severe.

Chapter 6

HYPOTHYROIDISM

HYPOTHYROIDISM is the physical disorder which results from too little thyroid hormone available in the body. The term "myxedema" may be employed synonymously with hypothyroidism, but more often is used to imply a particularly severe degree of hypothyroidism. Most of the hypothyroidism seen in the United States at this time is the result of previous thyroid surgery or radiation therapy. A smaller, but significant number of people develop hypothyroidism as a result of inflammatory disease, e.g. Hashimoto's thyroiditis, or subacute thyroiditis (see Chapter 9). Finally, there are a number of rare conditions which lead to impaired thyroid hormone synthesis, or thyroid tissue destruction. Regardless of the cause or mechanism of the hypothyroidism, the picture produced is dependent primarily upon the severity of the thyroid hormone deficiency.

Symptoms of Hypothyroidism

Hypothyroid patients complain of loss of memory, and decreased intellectual capacity. There are muscle cramps, numbness of the arms and legs (falling asleep), the sensation of being cold all the time, decreased hearing, husky voice, dry coarse skin, heavy and prolonged menstrual periods, and constipation. The patient will admit to fatigue, but it is more than the fatigue which is so common in the neurotic middleaged woman. The hypothyroid patient actually sleeps excessively, often napping for an hour or two, two or three times during the day, as well as sleeping all night. The fatigue syndrome in neurosis is usually associated with decreased sleeping, even difficulty in falling asleep.

Findings on Examination of Hypothyroid Patients

The physical examination reveals a patient with puffiness of the face, particularly under the eyes (Fig. 15). The skin has a yellow cast and is dry, flaky, and thickened. The voice is deep. The hair is coarse and lifeless. Tapping of the muscle tendons with the reflex hammer produces a very sluggish response. The patient may even fall asleep during the interview or examination if the disorder is severe. The pulse is slow, usually less than seventy beats per minute. Goiter is commonly present.

Laboratory Tests in Hypothyroidism

Laboratory tests show decreased thyroid hormone levels in the blood and a decreased uptake of radioactive iodine by the thyroid gland. The results of laboratory tests in hypothyroidism have been outlined in Chapter 3. To summarize, the FTI is low, the T_3(RIA) is low, the TSH(RIA) is elevated, and the RAI uptake is low and fails to respond normally to TSH simulation.

These are the findings for the vast majority of hypothyroid patients for whom the disorder is one affecting the thyroid gland itself. Rarely, the difficulty is within the pituitary gland, impairing its ability to release thyroid-stimulating hormone (TSH). This possibility is suggested if there is evidence of pituitary tumor with or without the suggestion of decreased function of other endocrine glands (principally the adrenal and ovaries or testes). If the patient has hypothyroidism on the basis of pituitary disease the TSH (RIA) will not be elevated, and there will be a normal response to the RAI uptake on a TSH stimulation test. It is important to recognize the rare patient with a pituitary disorder, for these patients treatment of the hypothyroidism without correction of a concurrent hypoadrenalism may prove disastrous.

Treatment of Hypothyroidism

The treatment of hypothyroidism is thyroid hormone. Figure 15 shows the change in appearance which occurred after treatment with thyroid hormone for two months.

There are a number of commercially available preparations but they are basically of two types. The more modern preparations are synthetic compounds, whereas the original preparations were crude products of animal origin (desiccated thyroid). For many years,

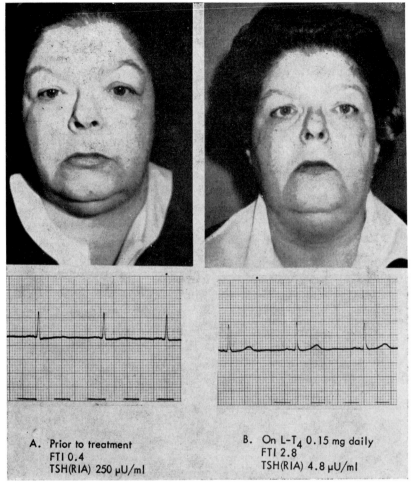

A. Prior to treatment
FTI 0.4
TSH(RIA) 250 µU/ml

B. On L-T₄ 0.15 mg daily
FTI 2.8
TSH(RIA) 4.8 µU/ml

FIGURE 15. A patient with hypothyroidism. A, Before treatment. Note the puffiness of the face. B, After treatment the appearance is much improved.

only the animal preparations were available. These prove quite satisfactory for most people. However, the quantity of active hormone in each pill, and in each batch of pills, may be variable. Occasional batches which are almost without potency continue to crop up. For these reasons, efforts have been expended to synthesize pure chemical thyroid hormone preparations which would be constant in potency. Such preparations are now available at very reasonable cost and are widely replacing the more crude products.

The average hypothyroid patient can be restored to complete normality (the euthyroid state) with relative ease in a matter of a few months once the diagnosis is established. Adequate treatment requires daily medication, but there is no reason to take thyroid hormone more than once daily, since thyroid hormone is very long acting. Convenient dosage sizes of the pure synthetic thyroid hormone are available so that only a single pill need be taken each day. There is no special time of day when this medication must be taken. Thyroid hormone is slow to produce its effects, and these effects last for a relatively long period of time (several weeks). Patients frequently report an improved sense of well-being immediately after taking the pill in the morning, and a prompt deterioration in their condition if a single pill is missed. Neither of these responses is possible in terms of body function. The thyroid hormone medication one takes today has its effect in about ten days, and that taken about ten days previously is responsible for today's health. One must stop thyroid hormone pills for about three weeks for all of the hormone to be used up by the body. Even then, the full-blown picture of hypothyroidism might not appear for several additional weeks. Bona fide hypothyroidism almost always requires treatment for life. Unfortunately patients frequently fail to take their medication faithfully. This is a particularly common problem with the older patient, who may lapse into an hypothyroid state over and over again if the administration of the medication is not closely supervised. Hypothyroidism, although completely correctable if diagnosed promptly and treated properly, may be lethal if uncorrected for a long enough period of time. The patient tends to become progressively lethargic, lapses into coma, and succumbs. The coma of hypothyroidism is extremely serious, and in spite of all available treatments, almost half these patients die.

Hypothyroidism in the Newborn

Hypothyroidism of the newborn, although rare, is an extremely serious illness. Unless promptly treated, growth retardation and permanent brain damage will result (cretin). Checking for hypothyroidism is one of the important services performed by the physician at the time of his initial examination of the newborn infant. The quantity of thyroid hormone required for treatment in infants and children is remarkably similar to that used for adults. In fact, after two or three years of age, full adult doses are employed.

Elderly Hypothyroid Patients

Treatment of the elderly hypothyroid patient may be particularly difficult. Forgetfulness is such a frequent problem that some of these patients lapse into hypothyroidism over and over, often becoming severely ill before the family realizes that the patient once again has not been taking his medication. Heart disease is a common complicating factor which limits the ability of the elderly hypothyroid to tolerate the very thyroid hormone for which his body is in such great need. These patients present some of the most complicated and difficult problems with which a physician must deal. In many instances, less than complete success must be accepted as the best compromise for a difficult situation.

Chapter 7

THYROID NODULES AND THYROID CANCER

"Nodule" is the term physicians apply to lumps between the size of about a pea, to those of a golf ball. The term is non-specific. Any kind of lump within these general size limitations can be called a nodule. Therefore, "nodule" is not really a diagnosis, but simply a descriptive term for a gross abnormality detected by physical examination, whose true nature can only be determined by further investigation. In the final analysis, removal of the nodule and microscopic examination of the tissue is the only means to provide final proof of the nature of the tissue. The most important concern for thyroid nodules is the possibility that they may harbor cancer.

Since breast nodules carry a rather high risk of fatal malignancy, most physicians encourage self-examination of the breast, and prompt removal of nodules detected in this fashion, or at the time of routine physical examination. With thyroid nodules the problem is vastly different. About 50 percent of the population over fifty years of age, and a lesser but still important proportion of the younger population, will have thyroid nodules. A moment's reflection makes it obvious that there are millions of people with this problem. Many, if not most of these people, proceed about their daily routines completely unaware of the presence of these lumps.

The vast majority of thyroid nodules are entirely benign, and many of those classified as malignant on the basis of microscopic examination cause no problems for the patients even when present for years. Yet a small proportion of thyroid nodules harbor thyroid cancers which can cause trouble, including even death in rare instances. It is these nodules which we wish to remove as soon as possible. Removal of all detected thyroid nodules, to be sure that every potentially dangerous nodule is eliminated, is an impractical and dangerous approach to the problem. There are not enough hospital beds, physicians, nursing, and other personnel available to begin to care for the vast number of patients with thyroid nodules, even if all available medical personnel and facilities were devoted solely to this problem. Furthermore, surgery on the thyroid gland, although very safe when performed by capable physicians, nevertheless is followed by minor to major complications in a significant proportion of patients. Therefore, if all thyroid nodules were to be removed, the number of patients who would suffer from the inevitable surgical complications, would far exceed the number who would actually benefit from the surgery. In other words, the cure would be worse than the disease. For this reason, most physicians advise removal of only those nodules which seem most likely to be malignant, and continued observation of the rest. The principle of selective surgery for thyroid nodules by and large works well in the hands of experienced physicians. Nevertheless, whenever an opinion must be offered, based upon judgment and experience, the wrong opinion will be given in some instances. The more experienced the physician, the fewer the errors. Perfection cannot be expected. Unfortunately, there is no better alternative. Medicine is not an exact science.

To make the determination of which thyroid nodules are best removed and which can be observed, the physician follows the same well-worn path he takes in the evaluation of any other medical problem—history, physicial examination, and laboratory tests.

History for Thyroid Nodule Patients

The younger the patient, the more likely is the nodule to be malignant. Benign nodules are frequent in older people, simply on the basis of wear and tear. The younger the patient, the less acceptable is this explanation. Furthermore if the patient is quite old, say in the sixties or seventies, the likelihood of a thyroid nodule harboring a surgically curable cancer, which, without surgery, would cause trouble for the patient is small. Most thyroid cancer follows a very sluggish course, growing very slowly and spreading only after many years. Hence, the older the patient, the less likely is the physician to advise surgery. The frequency of thyroid nodules which arises on the basis of benign disease is much less in men than in women. Therefore, a nodule in a man is usually regarded with greater suspicion.

Recently it has been shown that previous x-ray therapy directed at tissues in the neck area may predispose to thyroid cancer. This was first recognized in patients who had received x-ray therapy for an enlarged thymus gland detected soon after birth. The thymus gland is a structure located in the fore part of the upper chest. In many newborn infants it is quite prominent, tending to regress spontaneously with the passage of time. Between twenty and thirty years ago, it was widely believed that an enlarged thymus gland could asphyxiate a baby by obstructing the windpipe. Since thymus tissue is quite sensitive to x-ray therapy, many infants were so treated. It is now appreciated that this treatment is not only unnecsssary but also dangerous. A large number of thyroid cancers have developed in patients so treated. Since the tumors seem to appear ten or more years after the treatment, it is understandable that this unfortunate relationship was not recognized until many thousands of infants had been treated. More recently it has been shown that x-ray treatments to the tonsils and adenoids, and even to the skin of the face or neck may occasionally be followed by the development of thyroid cancer. Whenever a lump is discovered in a young person, a history of previous x-ray therapy makes thyroid cancer a very important consideration.

Findings on Physical Examination

The consistency of the nodule on physical examination is quite important. Cancers are usually very hard. Benign nodules feel much softer, even cystic. Cancers often appear to extend into adjacent tissue and may not be freely movable, as would be expected with a benign nodule. The presence of additional abnormal lumps in the neck outside the thyroid gland suggests early spread from a cancer rather than a benign nodule. These are a few of the important points which help the physician make his decision after the physical examination.

LABORATORY TESTS FOR THE EVALUATION OF THYROID NODULES

The Scan

The most important test which is employed to assist in the evaluation of thyroid nodules for malignant potential is the thyroid scan. As illustrated in Chapter 2, the thyroid scan is a pictorial representation of the iodine concentrating function of the thyroid tissue. The patient takes a small dose of radioactive iodine the day before the scan, and the scanning machine will detect and record the distribution of the iodine concentrated by the thyroid gland. Thyroid cancers concentrate iodine very poorly. If the location of the nodule is outlined carefully on the thyroid scan, one can compare the relative function of the nodule with that of the remaining presumably normal thyroid tissue. If the function of the nodule appears similar to that of the normal thyroid tissue, the likelihood of cancer is greatly reduced. On the contrary, if there is less than normal function in the nodule (hypofunctional nodule), the scan pattern is seen with thyroid cancer. Hypofunctional nodules may also be benign. In fact, only about 10 to 15 percent of hypofunctional nodules removed surgically prove to be malignant. Hence, the scan cannot be accepted as proof positive of cancer regardless of the picture; but if the nodule can be shown to be functional on scanning, the scan provides strong evidence against malignancy. In summary, scanning evidence of good function in a nodule reduces concern for cancer, evidence of less than normal function, although the usual finding in thyroid cancer, does not exclude a benign nodule.

Figure 16 is a composite of two thyroid scans which demonstrate nodules which have less function than normal thyroid tissue. In scan A of Figure 16 the thyroid nodule proved to be a cancer. The nodule shown in scan B of Figure 16 was a benign cyst. Nevertheless, the two nodules appear similar on scanning.

Figure 17 is an example of a clearly functional nodule in the left lobe of the thyroid gland. This nodule was benign. However, the lump on the right side of the neck was a thyroid cancer which had spread from a tiny focus of tumor in the right lobe of the thyroid gland, too small to show on the scan. The patient had received x-ray therapy for acne of the face fifteen years previously.

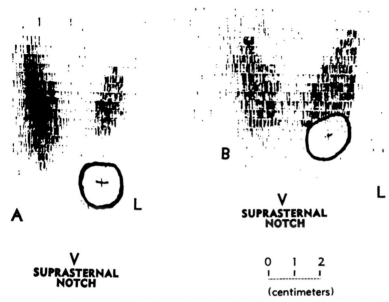

FIGURE 16. Two scans which show hypofunctional nodules. The circles have been placed on the scans by the doctor who monitored the test to show the locations of the margins of the nodules, in relation to the normally functioning thyroid tissue which can be seen without any marking because of its concentration of RAI. Since the nodules in these patients do *not* function, and thus do not concentrate RAI, the locations can only be determined on the basis of physical examination at the time the scan is done, and appropriate marking on the scan by the physician performing the examination. The nodule in scan A was malignant, however that in scan B was benign.

Ultrasound

As indicated in Chapter 3 diagnostic ultrasound will differentiate cystic from solid nodules. Figure 18 shows a patient with a nodule which is hypofunctional on scanning. The ultrasound tracing shows that it is solid (C of Fig. 18). The surgical specimen reveals a low-grade malignant tumor (D of Fig. 18).

Miscellaneous Tests

Other laboratory tests may offer assistance by providing data favoring diagnoses other than thyroid cancer, and are frequently employed.

To Take It Out or to Leave It In, that Is the Question

Finally, having completed the history and physical examination,

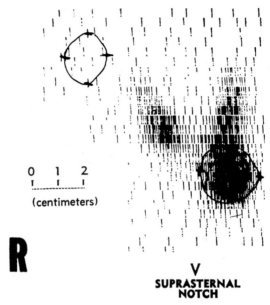

0   1   2

(centimeters)

R

V
**SUPRASTERNAL
NOTCH**

FIGURE 17. The scan shows an encircled functional nodule in the left lobe of the thyroid. This was benign. The encircled mass on the right was cancer which had spread into lymph nodes in the neck from a tumor of the right lobe, too small to feel.

and having obtained the appropriate laboratory tests, the physician is in a position to weigh the possibility of thyroid cancer against the risks of surgery, and finally to render a judgment as to the safest course of action for each patient. It should be obvious that this must be a personal, individual service. Rarely, if ever, does the physician encounter two patients with exactly similar situations. Just consider for a moment, all of the individual points which must be assessed with regard to the thyroid nodule itself. Then, one must still consider the general health of the patient in terms of past illness, and any current coincidental disorder. Is it any wonder then, that the physician is likely to throw up his hands in despair when the patient says, "But doctor, my friend has the very same thing, and his doctor advised an entirely different treatment!" Patients must accept the fact that medical problems which seem very simple to them may, in fact, have exceedingly complex ramifications. The physician must try to make the best judgment, not only for the moment, but also for the foreseeable future. Although the final rec-

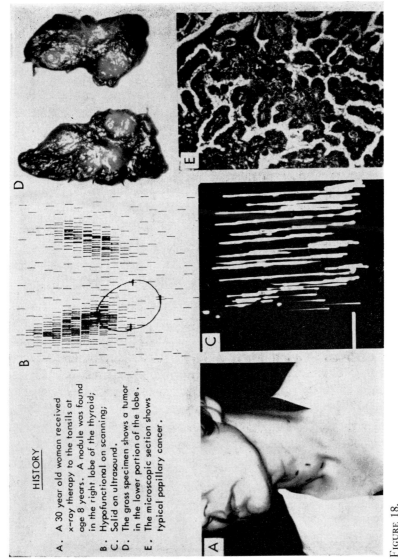

HISTORY

A. A 30 year old woman received x-ray therapy to the tonsils at age 8 years. A nodule was found in the right lobe of the thyroid;

B. Hypofunctional on scanning;

C. Solid on ultrasound.

D. The gross specimen shows a tumor in the lower portion of the lobe.

E. The microscopic section shows typical papillary cancer.

FIGURE 18.

ommendation may be only the simple phrase: "Take it out," or "Leave it in," the thought processes behind this advice is unbelievably complex. The physician's brain, acting much like a computer, compares all the available information on a particular patient with all his experience with similar cases in the past, and all the information he has obtained from his previous training and his continuing-study program. The judgments of experienced physicians have proved remarkably accurate in the evaluation of thyroid nodules for cancer.

TYPES OF THYROID CANCER

There are three basic types of thyroid cancer. They differ in terms of the age of the patient and the seriousness of the disease, hence some discussion is needed.

Anaplastic Thyroid Cancer

This is an uncommon form of thyroid cancer, involving less than ten percent of all thyroid cancer patients. It is almost never seen in patients less than forty years old, and most patients with this disease are older than sixty years. It is a very malignant condition. Almost all patients die within one year after the diagnosis is established. Some will benefit temporarily from x-ray treatment.

Medullary Thyroid Cancer

This form of cancer is also relatively uncommon. Sometimes it occurs in many members of the same family. Recently it has been possible to diagnose this disease with great precision by testing for the presence in the blood of a substance called calcitonin. Calcitonin may be detected on a blood test before there is any other evidence of cancer. Therefore, it is recommended that relatives of patients with medullary thyroid cancer be checked for calcitonin routinely. It is important to diagonose this disease as early as possible, for this increases the chances for cure. Medullary cancer is not as highly malignant as the anaplastic type, but is more dangerous than the differentiated forms to be discussed next.

Differentiated Forms of Thyroid Cancer

This category includes cancers termed either papillary or follicular on the basis of the microscopic appearance. They are found commonly in young people, and the younger the patient, the better the outlook. Patients under the age of forty years are almost always cured, and many older patients do well also. In fact, it may be said that if one has to have cancer, and has his choice as to the type, there are few that would be preferable to differentiated thyroid cancer.

Treatment of Thyroid Cancer

The treatment of thyroid cancer is primarily surgical. The surgeon attempts to remove all of the tumor tissue possible and in many cases the normal thyroid tissue as well. Thyroid cancers are often present in more than one part of the gland, and every bit of tumor may not be visible with the naked eye. Hence, removal of the entire thyroid offers additional assurance that there will be no recurrence. These cancers frequently extend outside the thyroid gland proper into the neck. It is very difficult to remove all of these extensions surgically. Fortunately, the remnants frequently will concentrate radioactive iodine (RAI) after the normal tissue is removed. This is true in spite of the fact that thyroid cancer tissue in general takes up RAI poorly. However, when competition by the normal thyroid tissue is eliminated by removing the thyroid gland, it is easier for any remaining cancer tissue to concentrate RAI. When this can be accomplished, a large dose of RAI will destroy the cancer tissue.

To permit any remaining thyroid cancer tissue to be stimulated to function maximally in terms of RAI concentration, no thyroid hormone is given for six weeks after surgery. During this period of time the blood thyroid hormone level in the patient falls, triggering the thyroid-pituitary feedback autoregulatory mechanism to cause a release of pituitary TSH, which in turn stimulates RAI uptake in any remaining thyroid tissue (normal or cancerous). Medication may also be given to enhance this process. Repeat scanning will permit the determination of whether or not there is residual cancer which can be treated with RAI. About 50 percent of thyroid cancer patients can benefit from treatment with RAI.

Following this testing period, and RAI therapy if needed, thyroid hormone is given to restore normal blood levels of thyroid hormone. This must be taken for life. These patients are usually checked yearly after the initial treatment is completed. The prognosis for thyroid cancer patients generally is excellent. In most instances, the survival rate of patients properly treated for thyroid cancer is similar to that for entirely normal people of the same age and sex.

Chapter 8

THYROID SURGERY

THYROID SURGEONS have contributed greatly over the years to the solution of thyroid problems. Newer concepts and techniques have served to focus more sharply the role of the surgeon for thyroid patients, but the importance of a well-trained and experienced surgeon has not been reduced.

INDICATIONS FOR THYROID SURGERY

1. Suspected thyroid cancer
2. Recurrent thyroid cancer
3. Hyperthyroidism
   a. Children not responding well to antithyroid drugs or with large, unsightly goiters
   b. Adults who prefer surgery to radioactive iodine
   c. Pregnant hyperthyroid patients who cannot tolerate antithyroid drugs
   d. Patients with toxic autonomously functioning thyroid nodules
4. Obstructing goiters
5. Unsightly goiters

The modern indications for thyroid surgery are outlined above. The most important and probably most common indication for surgery is a nodule which is suspicious for thyroid cancer. Also, about 10 percent of patients treated surgically for thyroid cancer may have a recurrent lump in the neck which must be removed at a later date.

Most hyperthyroid patients are treated successfully without surgery these days. However, there are exceptions. Children with large goiters often do not respond well to antithyroid drugs. Most physicians do not like to use radioactive iodine in growing children. Thus, the surgeon is called upon under these circumstances. Similarly, there is an occasional adult who prefers surgery to radioactice iodine. Pregnant hyperthyroid patients are usually treated with antithyroid drugs until after delivery. Then radioactive iodine can be given. However, if toxic reactions occur from the antithyroid drugs it may be necessary to advise surgery. Patients with hyperthyroidism from an autonomously functioning thyroid nodule may be treated with radioactive iodine, but the doses required are quite large, and therefore if the patient is young (i.e. less than forty years old) surgery may be preferable.

Very large goiters which produce obstruction to the trachea or esophagus, or simply are unsightly, are often best treated surgically.

WHAT SHOULD THE PATIENT EXPECT FROM THE SURGICAL EXPERIENCE?

A recommendation for thyroid surgery is often received by the patient with some degree of apprehension, and occasionally with outright panic. For some patients the idea of an operation on the neck is particularly frightening. Therefore let me say right now that it is not really so bad. In fact a thyroidectomy performed in a modern hospital by an experienced thyroid surgeon results in minimal discomfort, only a short hospital stay, and little risk of complication.

The Preliminary Visit with the Surgeon

The first step is to have a consultation with a surgeon. He will examine you and make the final determination as to whether surgery is necessary and likely to be beneficial. He will discuss with you the purpose of the surgery and its risks; and if you agree to proceed he will make a reservation for you with the hospital. Hyperthyroid patients will have to take antithyroid pills for a period of four to six weeks (in most cases) to restore them to a state of normal thyroid function prior to surgery. The surgeon will want these medications continued up to the day of surgery. In addition he will order iodine drops for about ten days prior to the operation. The iodine drops serve to reduce the size of the goiter and to decrease chances for excessive bleeding during the surgery. It is very important that both of these medications be taken faithfully to assure a smooth and uncomplicated operation.

Patients who do not have hyperthyroidism seldom require any special preparation for thyroid surgery.

The Hospital Stay

Preparation for Surgery

The duration of hospitalization for the usual patient requiring thyroid surgery is less than one week. In some cases the patient need only stay three or four days. At times it is necessary to be in the hospital for a few days before the surgery is done to correct or improve any problem which might increase the risk of surgery. For example, if the patient happens to have a weak heart showing signs of failure, it might be desirable to check this further, and correct it as far as possible under the closer observation which can be pursued in the hospital.

The day before surgery the anesthesiologist will visit with you and discuss the plans for anesthesia. Methods of anesthesia may have to be tailored individually to the patient's needs if there are any other illnesses or a history of drug sensitivity. A house physician also will perform a final examination to make sure that nothing has occurred which might make it necessary to alter plans for surgery. These checks and double checks may seem annoying, but you should remember that they are done for your protection. Therefore cooperate and make the best of it.

The night before surgery you will be given medication to assure a good night's sleep. The next morning you will also receive medication to make you drowsy and prepare you for the anesthesia. You will be taken to the surgical section and again meet the anesthesiologist. You may not see your surgeon, for quite likely he will be busy elsewhere until you are asleep and ready for him to get on with his job. The anesthesiologist will say a few words to you while an intravenous solution is started. This involves inserting a small needle into one of your veins. It will cause no real discomfort. In a few moments you will be asleep.

The Operation

The surgeon will begin the operation by making an incision across the neck. If you look at your neck you will notice that there are a number of horizontal lines or creases in the skin. The surgeon attempts to make the incision in one of these creases to minimize any visible scarring. The incision is usually about three to four inches long. From the skin the surgeon proceeds through various muscles and other tissues down to the thyroid. How much thyroid tissue is removed depends upon the reason for the surgery and the extent of the disease. Sometimes half the thyroid, and sometimes all must be removed. The usual duration of the operation is about two hours.

After the surgery is completed you will be taken to the recovery room where specially trained nurses will check you until the anesthesia has worn off and you are in condition to return to your room.

The pain from thyroid surgery is usually much less than patients expect. Ordinarily the patient is out of bed the evening of the surgery, and able to eat and receive visitors. Within forty-eight hours there is seldom any need for pain medication. The scar itself takes up to one year for complete healing and for all of the redness to disappear.

After Care

Following release from the hospital in most instances the patient can resume full activities within a few days. If the surgery was for hyperthyroidism, it will be necessary to have further testing periodically to determine whether thyroid hormone tablets are needed. It may also be desirable to have the blood calcium levels checked for reasons to be discussed shortly. If the surgery was for a thyroid nodule or large obstructing goiter, thyroid hormone tablets will be needed to prevent a recurrent nodular goiter from forming—even if the surgeon believes that there is enough normal thyroid tissue remaining to produce all the thyroid hormone the patient may need (see below). In addition to any examination performed soon after the surgery, an annual checkup is desirable to assure that thyroid (if needed) is being taken in proper dosage, and to rule out any changes in the status of the remaining thyroid tissue which might indicate the need for further testing or evaluation.

COMPLICATIONS OF THYROIDECTOMY

Thyroid surgery is much safer now than it has ever been in the past. However no surgery is risk-free. In fact, a very important part of the decision to recommend surgery is based upon an evaluation of the risk of the surgery, compared to the risks of the disease. Only if the disease seems to carry the greater risk is surgery advised. Since risks are unavoidable they must be discussed.

The risk which is of most concern to most patients is death. It is a fact of life that some patients do not survive surgery, and thyroid surgery is no exception. To be sure, the risk of death is very small. There are reports from leading hospitals which cover up to one thousand consecutive thyroid operations without a single death. On the other hand most hospitals in which sizable numbers of patients have thyroid surgery, do report an occasional fatality. These catastrophes are seldom related to the surgery itself. Sometimes it is an unexpected complication of the anesthesia, or the result of an unexpected and unavoidable cardiac complication. With all of the modern techniques available to check and double check patients prior to thyroid surgery the chances of an unexpected fatality are becoming less and less. Certainly the risk is so small that it need not deter one from having necessary surgery.

Thyroid surgery has certain special risks because of the location of the thyroid gland. The thyroid lies over the larynx (voice box). The nerves which control voice lie very close to the thyroid gland, and some may even pass through it. Therefore thyroid surgery always has the risk of unavoidable injury to these nerves, which could cause an impairment of voice. Singing voice is frequently affected. Spoken voice is less commonly impaired (probably no more than 1 to 2 percent of patients have this problem).

The parathyroids (there are four usually) are small glands which lie right next to the thyroid gland. These have the function of controlling the blood calcium level. They may inadvertently be removed during thyroid surgery, or if not removed may be injured or their blood supply impaired so that sooner or later they are unable to function. Should this happen the blood calcium level will fall. If unrecognized and uncorrected this can lead to cataracts, seizures and calcification of vital portions of the brain. These problems will be prevented if the blood calcium level is checked periodically and subnormal levels corrected with medication. Calcium supplements alone may be all that is need. It is important that calcium not be taken with food, for this will reduce its availability to the body. Occasionally vitamin D supplements may be needed. Vitamin D should be taken only under careful medical supervision, for an excessive amount may produce a harmful elevation in blood calcium levels.

Most patients do require replacement doses of thyroid hormone after thyroid surgery. There are two reasons for which thyroid hormone might be needed. First, there may be too little remaining thyroid tissue to produce all the thyroid hormone needed for the body. Second, even if a sizable amount of thyroid tissue is left behind, it may tend to enlarge or become nodular if no thyroid hormone is given. This happens because a part of the thyroid gland will be asked to do the job of a whole thyroid. It may not be able to do it without enlarging, and in the course of enlarging may develop lumps. This is easily prevented by taking thyroid hormone. One pill a day is all that is necessary, and the cost is only about ten dollars per year.

There are other lesser complications of thyroid surgery, including infections or bleeding from the wound, an unsightly scar and a host of minor annoyances. However, these do not require a lengthy discussion. Some comment might be needed with reference to the scar. All experienced surgeons attempt to close a thyroidectomy incision just as a plastic surgeon would, for they want the patient to have the finest scar possible. However, the final result is not entirely under the control of the surgeon. Some patients just heal badly. Occasionally further repairative surgery may help correct the scar, but some patients will have to accept the fact that it may be necessary to live with a scar which is unattractive.

Chapter 9

THYROIDITIS

WHENEVER ONE ENCOUNTERS the ending "itis" on a word it is safe to conclude that there is reference to inflammation. Therefore, thyroiditis is a disease characterized by inflammation. Inflammation is a defensive reaction of the body to any kind of tissue injury. The reaction takes the form of an invasion of the area of injury by specialized blood cells which have the capability of fighting infection and promoting healing.

Subacute Thyroiditis

One of the more common types of thyroiditis is called "subacute" thyroiditis because the patient is generally not very ill. This condition is thought to be the result of infection by any of several types of viruses. Pain, tenderness and swelling in the region of the thyroid gland are the hallmarks of subacute thyroiditis. There is usually a slight to moderate fever. The patient often complains of weakness, lack of pep and energy, and sometimes generalized aches and pains. As a result of destruction of tissue by the invading virus, stored thyroid hormone may be released into the blood in larger than normal quantities. This can produce a temporary mild hyperthyroid state.

Laboratory tests of value in confirming the diagnosis of subacute thyroiditis include an elevated white blood count (the white blood cells combat infection), an increase in the blood sedimentation rate (a nonspecific indicator of inflammation), elevated levels by tests which measure blood thyroid hormone levels (for reasons cited above), and a very low RAI uptake (because the ability of thyroid tissue to concentrate iodine is temporarily impaired by the widespread inflammation). The diagnosis of subacute thyroiditis is rather simple when the patient has the characteristic symptoms, physical examination findings, and laboratory tests values. However, the severity and extent of the disease may vary greatly. In very mild cases the symptoms may be limited to just a general feeling of illness with perhaps a slight discomfort in the neck area. The usual laboratory tests may be normal or so slightly altered that no diagnosis can be established. When the symptoms are minimal there may not even be a medical consultation. In some instances an incorrect diagnosis of influenza or a simple upper respiratory infection may be made. Fortunately, spontaneous recovery within a few weeks is the rule, regardless of diagnosis or treatment. When the involvement is more severe, treatment by a physician becomes necessary. Although antibiotics (drugs to kill bacteria) have frequently been employed for subacute thyroiditis, there is no evidence that they are of any value. The usual treatment includes aspirin and simple medications for pain relief. If the pain is unusually severe or prolonged it may be necessary to administer cortisone-like drugs, and even x-ray therapy. In some instances the disease may run a protracted course over several months, punctuated by repeated flare-ups. Ultimately, even in these patients, there is usually complete recovery. However, there may be a residual hypothyroidism (resulting from failure of recovery of function), goiter (compensatory in types, resulting from impaired function—see Chapter 4), or both.

Thus, subacute thyroiditis may be an annoying little illness even though there are usually no serious consequences.

Acute Thyroiditis

Much less common is the acute form of thyroiditis, caused by bacterial infection. (There is some confusion in the terminology physicians use for thyroiditis. Some call more severe forms of what has been described as "subacute thyroiditis," "acute thyroiditis." But the preferred usage is to limit the designation "acute" to the rare bacterial form.) These patients are severely ill with high fever and evidence of abscess formation in the neck. The overlying skin is reddened, hot and exquisitely tender to the touch. Acute thyroiditis is a medical emergency requiring intensive treatment with antibiotics and surgical drainage. Without prompt attention it is possible to die from this disorder. Although acute thyroiditis has been a very rare occurrence in the past, the increased illegal use of drugs is leading to a significant increase in this problem. Drug addicts frequently try to inject materials directly into the large veins of the neck with improperly sterilized equipment (if indeed any effort at cleanliness is made). Accidentally piercing the thyroid gland can lead to infection.

Hashimoto's Disease

One of the more common causes of inflammatory goiter is Hashimoto's disease, a form of chronic thyroiditis named in honor of the Japanese physician who described the condition. The patient usually has a characteristic woody-hard goiter and a variable degree (usually mild) of hypothyroidism. Although this disease is most common in the middle-aged woman, recently it has been appreciated that Hashimoto's disease is one of the more common causes of goiter in children. Treatment with thyroid hormone is generally all that is required. This treatment must be maintained for life. At times the goiter may be nodular, and in some instances surgery may be necessary to rule out cancer. For patients with Hashimoto's disease who have part of the thyroid removed, subsequent treatment with thyroid hormone is particularly important. This treatment will not only assure that there are adequate supplies of this essential substance, but also prevent the development of compensatory goiter by the remaining tissue.

Riedel's Struma

An exceedingly rare form of thyroiditis is known as Riedel's struma (Struma is the German word for goiter). In this disease normal thyroid tissue is replaced by a pale white tough sinewy material (fibrous tissue) which may extend beyond the confines of the thyroid gland causing adherence to adjacent tissues. As the process extends there may be compression of the trachea (windpipe), even to the point of asphyxiation. The only treatment is surgical. The cause of this disease is unknown.

Traumatic Thyroiditis?

Whether physical trauma can produce a true inflammatory reaction in the thyroid gland remains controversial. The increasing frequency of injury to soft tissues of the neck resulting from automobile accidents has led to a reconsideration of the possibility of traumatic thyroiditis. Needless to say, the legal implications of this diagnosis are far reaching. Although some of the patients who complain of neck pain following auto accidents are motivated by visions of large insurance settlements, we have seen an occasional victim of neck trauma who did have what appeared to be objective evidence of temporary injury to the thyroid gland. However, the frequency of such an injury must be quite small.

Chapter 10

THYROID FUNCTION— MENSTRUATION, FERTILITY AND PREGNANCY

PHYSICIAN UNDERSTANDING of the relationship of thyroid function to menstruation, fertility, and pregnancy, has left much to be desired. Availability of relatively potent thyroid hormone preparations was preceded by many years full knowledge of their proper use. Lacking any other effective treatment, and in view of the relative safety of small doses of thyroid hormone in young people, thousands of women with menstrual irregularities or infertility routinely have been given thyroid hormone. Pregnant women also have received this drug, almost as one might employ a "tonic." Much of this unwarranted and improper treatment has been justified by inaccurate basal metabolic rate (BMR) determinations. It is now clear that unless there is bona fide hypothyroidism, thyroid hormone is worthless in these situations. The frequency with which thyroid hormone is used without justification is dropping remarkably as physicians are becoming more aware of the proper indications for this medication.

Menstrual Abnormalities

Nevertheless, both hypothyroidism and hyperthyroidism do affect menstruation, fertility, and pregnancy. In hypothyroidism the menstrual periods tend to be prolonged and heavy, while the hyperthyroid patient usually has scanty periods. Correction of abnormal thyroid function leads to restoration of normal cycles in both instances. Any abnormality of thyroid function reduces fertility, but when thyroid function is normal, the use of thyroid hormone for infertility is worthless.

Fertility

Pregnancy is difficult to achieve when thyroid function is abnormal. However, if the woman does become pregnant and is hypothyroid, miscarriage or damage to the fetus is quite likely. Hyperthyroidism, unless severe, is less dangerous to both mother and fetus. Pregnancy tends to reduce the severity of hyperthyroidism. Treatment of the pregnant hyperthyroid patient is usually satisfactorily accomplished with antithyroid drugs. It is important to avoid overtreatment, for this will result in hypothyroidism and probably fetal damage. Large quantities of iodine should not be given to the pregnant hyperthyroid patient, for this may lead to impairment of function of the fetal thyroid gland, with the development of a large goiter, and brain damage. Thyroidectomy has been advised frequently in the past for the pregnant hyperthyroid patient. Since major surgery on the pregnant woman poses a significant risk to the fetus, this method of management is becoming less popular. After pregnancy is terminated, the treatment of the mother is pursued just as it would have been had she not been pregnant, with the exception that radioactive iodine may not be given if she is nursing the baby. The radioactive iodine would be secreted into the mother's milk and could injure the infant's thyroid.

Neonatal Hyperthyroidism

Rarely, the offspring of a hyperthyroid mother will develop hyperthyroidism in the first few days of life. Very recently it has been shown that this is caused by a transfer from the mother to the baby of an abnormal thyroid-stimulating substance which stimulates the baby's thyroid to function excessively. It usually takes three to four weeks for this substance to disappear and normal thyroid function to be restored. During this interval the hyperthyroidism can usually be controlled by the addition of iodine drops to the formula.

Chapter 11

COMMON FICTIONS ABOUT THE THYROID GLAND AND ITS FUNCTIONS

BECAUSE CRUDE, BUT EFFECTIVE, thyroid hormone preparations in pill form have been available for many years; because the administration of this hormone in small doses is, with rare exception, harmless; and finally, because in the hypothyroid patient thyroid hormone may produce a dramatic restoration of health and vigor, thyroid hormone has historically enjoyed wide use, often for the slimmest reasons, and even in the absence of a valid reason. Primarily as the result of this misuse of thyroid hormone and secondarily as an outgrowth of a desire on the part of both patient and physician for quick and simple solutions to either difficult or impossible problems, a body of misinformation on the value of thyroid hormone has gained acceptance as fact by laymen, and in some instances, even by physicians. Some of the more common of these misconceptions will be discussed.

Obesity Is Commonly Caused by Hypothyroidism

It is true that some hypothyroid patients are obese, but not all. Some patients with hypothyroidism are slender. For the hypothyroid individual, as for all other persons, obesity is a result of eating more food than the body needs. For the obese hypothyroid individual, as for all other obese people, weight reduction is impossible without sustained caloric restriction.

Hypothyroidism is never the sole cause of severe obesity. Obesity is a common condition in all developed areas of the world, and is

78

especially common in the United States, yet hypothyroidism is a distinctly uncommon disorder. Extensive testing of obese patients to rule out possible hypothyroidism, although widely done because of the intense lay prejudice for the misconception of hypothyroidism as a cause of obesity, is generally a wasteful procedure. Less than one obese patient in one thousand will have hypothyroidism as even a contributing factor in the weight gain. Yet, it is a rare obese patient indeed who has not been given thyroid hormone at some time, in a vain effort at restoring the patient to normal weight. Thyroid hormone is one of the components of the notorious "diet pills" which have resulted in the death of a number of patients, yet are still being consumed in vast quantities by an uninformed and unsuspecting public.

Overweight children are commonly sent to me with a diagnosis of hypothyroidism. They seldom have it. There are two easily assessed points which help to indicate the likelihood of hypothyroidism. Overfed children are tall, hypothyroid children are short. Hypothyroid children usually have goiter, if they are not obvious cretins. Therefore, a tall obese child without goiter is very unlikely to have hypothyroidism.

This problem of obesity will be discussed in greater detail in Chapter 12.

The "Tired Housewife" Is a Victim of Hypothyroidism

One of the most common complaints with which the physician must deal is "fatigue." The patient is usually a female, between thirty and sixty years of age. She is just as tired when she gets up in the morning as when she retires at night. By midmorning she feels somewhat better, but by late afternoon, she is really "pooped" and just "drags around" until bedtime. Paradoxically, she does not sleep well. Either she has trouble falling asleep, or awakens after only four to six hours of sleep, and cannot get back to sleep. Occasionally, more severe insomnia is present. As the condition becomes worse, she becomes unable to keep up with her household duties, even neglects her personal appearance. There are crying spells and withdrawal from social contacts. Gloomy thoughts preoccupy her mind. The diagnosis of a psychoneurotic depression at this point is quite simple. In most instances, the condition is present in rather mild form, and the principal or sole symptom is fatigue ("I am tired all the time.") She is bored with routine duties or perhaps temporarily overburdened with responsibilities, all seeming to crush in upon her at once, with no respite in sight.

The precise circumstances and events capable of precipitating this complaint of fatigue are as varied as it is possible to imagine. Fortunately, most patients overcome these episodes without great difficulty. However, as the problem runs its course, many patients find their way to the endocrinologist, convinced by self, or well-meaning friends, neighbors, or relatives, that a bad thyroid gland is at the bottom of the trouble. It is true that a deficiency of thyroid hormone can cause fatigue, but it is a far different type of symptom from that just described. The hypothyroid patient is not only tired, but somnolent. He sleeps all night and a good part of the day, as well. Not only is there physical fatigue but mental lethargy as well. Mistakes in business or household activities are common. Extensive forgetfulness is characteristic. In addition, there are other symptoms of hypothyroidism previously described in Chapter 6. Interestingly enough, the true hypothyroid patient often fails even to mention fatigue as a symptom. More likely are complaints of muscle cramps, numbness, cold intolerance, facial puffiness, or hoarseness. The physician must ask about the excessive sleeping to discover that it is part of the picture.

Mental Deficiency Is Commonly Caused by Hypothyroidism

Every physician sooner or later encounters the pathetic anguished mother with a retarded child, hoping against hope that there is a solution for the problem, if only the right doctor will think of the right medicine. ("Maybe his thyroid is a little off, Doctor?") Of course, thyroid deficiency may cause severe mental retardation in the infant, if uncorrected. Unfortunately, once the damage is done no correction is possible. One of the most important services performed by the physician as part of the newborn checkup is to exclude the possibility of hypothyroidism. Only a minute fraction of the mentally retarded population of the United States is the result of thyroid deficiency.

Short Stature Is Commonly the Result of Hypothyroidism

Again, it is true that children who are deficient in thyroid hormone will fail to achieve their full growth potential. However, of all the short people, the proportion with hypothyroidism as a cause of their lack of growth is so small as to be negligible. The vast majority of short people are simply the product of short parents or parents who transmit hereditary factors producing short stature. It is just as inevitable that some of us will be short, as that some will be tall. Why our culture places such emphasis on height, especially for males, is difficult to understand, especially if one considers the outstanding contributions of the shorter individuals. In any event, unless short stature is accompanied by the other manifestations of hypothyroidism, extensive thyroid testing is futile.

Thinning Hair Means Thyroid Deficiency

Again, it is true that patients with hypothyroidism, and also hyperthyroidism, tend to lose hair excessively and that correction of the thyroid disorder leads to a restoration of hair growth. However, the hair loss associated with thyroid disease never occurs as an isolated phenomenon. There are always other findings which point to the true nature of the disorder. Hair loss not accompanied by other findings of thyroid disease, and particularly a patchy hair loss (alopecia areata), or total hair loss (alopecia totalis) is not due to thyroid disease, and cannot be improved by the thyroid hormone.

Thyroid Disease Is a Major Cause of Infertility

Patients with either hypothyroidism, or hyperthyroidism, have reduced fertility, particularly when the disorder is severe. But these conditions are easily recognized and corrected. Therefore, the likelihood of an infertile patient, particularly if without evidence of thyroid disease, benefiting from an investigation of thyroid gland function, or treatment directed at the thyroid gland, is extremely remote. Nevertheless, primarily because of the availability of thyroid hormone and the lack of other specific remedies, thyroid hormone pills by the millions have been consumed in the vain hope of achieving conception.

Hypofunctional ("Cold") Thyroid Nodules Are Usually Malignant

When thyroid scanning became possible, it was hoped that the differences in the ability to concentrate radioactive iodine would permit differentiation of benign and malignant thyroid nodules. For some time it had been known that thyroid cancer appeared to have little of the functional characteristics of normal thyroid tissue; and sure enough from the very beginning of scanning, it was noted that malignant thyroid nodules concentrated radioactive iodine very poorly. The terms "cold," or more recently "hypofunctional," have been applied to these nodules. This is in contrast to nodules which have function approximately equivalent to that of normal tissue ("warm") or increased function ("hot"). Nodules with as much or greater function than normal thyroid tissue (in terms of concentration of radioactive iodine) are probably never malignant. Since malignant nodules are almost always hypofunctional, and functional nodules are almost always benign, the concept that hypofunctional nodules are usually malignant was quickly disseminated into the medical literature, and remains riveted into the minds even of physicians. This line of reasoning is about as sound as the following: Gold glitters; material which fails to glitter is seldom, if ever, gold; therefore, all that glitters is gold.

Lack of experience with newer techniques employing radioactive tracer materials has led to confusion in the minds of physicians who on more familiar ground are exceedingly able and sophisticated. As previously discussed in Chapter 7, anything which impairs the function of a portion of the thyroid gland will produce an area of hypofunction on scanning. This includes degeneration, inflammation, hemorrhage, and benign as well as malignant tumors. Thyroid nodules are extremely common, whereas thyroid cancer is very rare. Most thyroid nodules are hypofunctional. In the author's experience with thousands of thyroid nodules, hypofunctional nodules predominate over functional at the rate of about three to one, yet of the hypofunctional group less than one in ten proves to be malignant. Scanning is of help in the determination of which thyroid nodules should be removed. However, the principal value of scanning is providing evidence of function in a nodule, thus relieving concern for malignancy. Varying degrees of reduced function must be correlated with the other features in the clinical picture.

Take Kelp for Good Health

One of the latest fads in food supplements is kelp. Many virtues are claimed for this material. These claims are almost completely false. There is only one type of thyroid problem which might benefit from kelp, and this is rare and more easily and more effectively treated with thyroid hormone. Kelp is simply seaweed, and contains a large amount of iodine. Iodized salt provides all the iodine you need. Excessive iodine intake may cause falsely abnormal thyroid function tests, and may aggravate minor thyroid defects to produce goiter and hypothyroidism.

Each of the above fictions has a kernel of truth upon which has been built a mountain of superstition, misinformation, and just plain gossip. If one could calculate the needless expense, wasted time and effort, false hopes, and ultimate disappointment which has resulted from the useless search for nonexistent hypothyroidism, and the worthless administration of thyroid hormone, the result would indeed be staggering. Since thyroid hormone is required for the proper function of every organ and tissue in the body, when deficient or present in excess, the resulting disorder produces a number of symptoms and alterations in the body detectable by physical examination. Isolated complaints, or physical findings are almost never the result or inadequate or excess thyroid hormone secretion.

Chapter 12

OBESITY

OBESITY IS ONE OF THE MOST IMPORTANT public health problems in the United States today. Life insurance statistics indicate that persons fifty pounds over their ideal weight have a one-third increase in mortality rate, and those with eighty pounds of excess weight have more than double the expected mortality rate. The obese have a higher incidence of diabetes mellitus, hypertension and coronary artery disease. Complications following elective or emergency surgery are more common. Beyond the physical disadvantages there are significant social problems. Opportunities for employment are limited, and so is the likelihood of advancement. Prospects for marriage are reduced, and the stability of an existing marriage may be impaired. The adverse effects of obesity are suffered not only by the overweight person himself, but they are also visited upon his children; for the offspring of the obese have a much greater probability of developing obesity.

Everyone agrees that obesity is bad, and that the overweight should reduce. Unfortunately the majority of obese people seem to be unable to achieve any sustained weight reduction.

Inevitably in the course of my daily activities as a thyroidologist, I see many patients for whom obesity is either the presenting complaint, or a prominent complicating factor. As a result, I have observed certain particularly common patterns of behavior and thinking which serve to deter the obese patient from realizing success with weight reduction.

THE EVOLUTION OF OBESITY

Recognizable obesity may have its onset at almost any time in life. It is common to obtain a history of onset when the child enters school, at adolescence, or following childbirth. Those who escape the obesity of early life are still subject to middle age spread or senescent obesity.

Many patients claim that they have been obese all their lives, and there is some truth in this attitude. An overprotective insecure mother may place undue emphasis upon eating. The infant soon learns that eating earns him a loving reward. In time, an altered setting of the central nervous system satiety center is produced so that only an excessive food intake proves satisfying. This may in part explain the observation that 75 percent of obese children maintain or increase their obesity as they grow into adulthood.

Regardless of the time of onset of obesity, psychological factors seem frequently to be operative. The overeating provides a real substitute for the fulfillment of needs that have not been met, and realistically are not likely to be met. Furthermore, the obese patient is subjected to continuing encouragement to persist in his eating by the advertising profession via radio, television and other media, which redundantly demonstrate the satisfactions to be achieved by indulging in food. Social situations place additional burdens upon the resolve of the obese patient as well-meaning friends and relatives encourage him to eat today and diet tomorrow. They do not realize how cruel this advice is to the struggling dieter. These powerful incentives to continue overeating compound the problem, and may render all efforts at correction unsuccessful.

Once a pattern of overeating has been established it tends to be perpetuated by certain characteristic habits and notions.

Faulty Habits

Obese individuals tend to fall into either of two categories with respect to eating habits.

Gross Overeating

The gross overeaters eat too much of all types of food at all meals, and in between as well. These constitute a minority of the obese patients seeking medical help. Gross overeating is either voluntary and deliberate, or the result of intellectual impairment or immaturity. For these patients there is neither regard nor concern for the consequences of their obesity and by and large they are content to pursue their faulty eating habits. At the behest of relatives, some of these patients may make an occasional half-hearted effort at weight reduction, but they seldom persist for very long. Probably best included with these patients are those whose obesity is the outward manifestation of a severe emotional disorder. Food has become so important and its deprivation so threatening that any meaningful attempt at weight reduction is impossible without a rather profound restructuring of the personality. My subsequent remarks exclude these gross overeaters. There is no effective, practical, and generally applicable approach to their management.

Overeating on Balance

The patient more likely to seek medical attention for obesity is not a gross overeater. It is a mistake to assume that all or even most obese patients are gluttons, in the usual sense of the word. In fact, many do not seem to be overeating at all, as we usually think of overeating. However, it is essential to define overeating apart from the usual stereotype of normalcy, which includes the concept of the balanced diet to which we were all exposed in grade school hygiene classes. Overeating simply means eating more food than the body needs. Note that the emphasis is upon body needs, not the quantity of food ingested per se. The excess intake of 3,500 calories will produce a weight gain of about one pound. Thus an average intake of 100 calories per day in excess of body needs may produce a ten pound weight gain per year, thirty pounds in three years, 100 pounds in ten years. One slice of bread, an apple, or five ounces of milk contain about 100 calories. No glutton worthy of the name would demean himself with such trivial overeating. Yet the consistent ingestion of even this amount of excess food may lead ultimately to obesity of monumental proportions.

This is not to imply that most obesity is the consequence of a small but regular excess intake, far from it. Much more common is the habit of periodic dieting punctuated by intermittent binges of varying length during which relatively enormous quantities of food may be consumed. In a single meal 3,000 or more calories may be ingested. These binges are often taken on weekends as rewards for faithful dieting during the week. The patient fails to appreciate that the rewards more than compensate for the prior caloric conservation and produce an overall positive caloric balance.

While dieting, the usual pattern of eating provides minimal caloric intake at breakfast and lunch, with a healthy supper, sometimes followed by evening snacks. Skipping breakfast and lunch only sharpens the appetite at supper, making it more difficult to curtail the intake, and easier to justify a larger meal than desirable. After all: "I haven't eaten all day." Furthermore, there is experimental evidence that this pattern of eating tends to promote a greater deposition of fat than would be the case with the ingestion of the same quantity of food, divided in three meals. These irregular eating habits make any attempt at an assessment of the average caloric content of the diet a very difficult undertaking.

Qualitative Aspects of Overeating

Qualitative factors in the diet also must be considered. Carbohydrates are converted into fat with less expenditure of energy than is the case for protein. Even a cursory investigation into the dietary habits of the obese commonly reveals a preference for bread, potatoes and other starches, not to mention sweets.

Physical Activity

In addition to faulty eating habits, lack of physical activity compounds the obesity problem. Many obese patients recognize their relative physical indolence. Others labor under the mistaken impression that they are very active, simply on the basis of routine household or business chores. To be sure this is a greater level of activity than bedrest; but to contribute significantly to a weight reduction program physical activity must be considerable and regular. For example, one hour of jogging consumes 600 calories; of swimming at a moderate rate, 500 calories; of cycling strenuously, 600 calories. By contrast, floor mopping, truck driving, ironing or food preparation utilize only about 200 calories per hour. Since the elimination of one pound of body fat necessitates the consumption of 3,500 calories, the following conclusions as to the role of physical activity in a weight reduction program seem justified:

1. To be useful, exercise must be regular, vigorous and prolonged;
2. One hour of vigorous exercise daily—every day—will result in the caloric consumption equivalent to one pound of fat per week;
3. Since most people are unable to exercise either so vigorously

or so regularly, exercise, although important, must be viewed as of supplemental value in a weight reduction program—for which caloric restriction is the keystone.

Faulty Notions

In addition to faulty habits, certain faulty notions manage to creep into the thinking of the obese individual and serve to inhibit efforts at corrective action.

Notions About Eating

"I really don't eat *that much*." "I have to starve myself to lose weight." "When I eat *normally* I gain." "I *have* to eat some bread or potatoes or I won't have a balanced diet." "I can gain ten pounds overnight!" *("Aren't you shocked, Doctor?")* "If I don't eat, I can't work." "I eat much less than my friend, and I gain while she stays thin." "I've tried every diet, and even if I lose a little at the beginning, I soon level off and sometimes even gain; so I just give up and go back to eating *normally*."

Note that there is some truth to each of these statements. As we have already seen, it is not necessary to eat "that much" to gain a considerable amount of weight. The concept of a "normal, balanced" diet as rooted in the lay mind is a distortion of fact and must be revised if progress with weight reduction is to be achieved. The most important element in this revision is an understanding of the nonessential nature of foods composed solely or predominantly of carbohydrates *(starches and sweets)*. One cannot only survive, but enjoy excellent health without them.

Obese patients frequently describe the disastrous weight gain which occurs when they eat "normally." Although eating "normally" surely means something quite specific to the patient, it means something quite different from patient to patient, and not very much at all to the physician. It is essential that the patient adjust his thinking to appreciate that what is normal for him, is no more than what is required to maintain a normal body weight. Therefore, by definition one who is obese, or gaining weight has not been, or is not, eating normally. The intake has exceeded body needs, and the excess calories have been stored as fat. Even if the patient does not eat "that much," it is too much for him.

Note the call for sympathy in the claim that "I must starve myself to lose," and the thinly veiled hostility in the statement "If I don't eat I can't work!" The patient knows she is not going to starve by dieting, and she knows that the doctor knows it. She does not have to be told that she has enough stored energy in her fat depots to do a great deal of work, even without eating, and can easily and safely carry on with a low caloric diet. These exaggerations simply reflect a desperate need for understanding and acceptance. They are frequently accompanied by a flow of tears expressing the underlying emotional intensity.

What obese patient has not tried dieting prior to consulting a physician? But what does she mean by trying, and what types of diets did she try? Trying may mean anything from a few days to a few weeks. When twenty pounds do not melt away the diet is considered a failure. If one asks the obese patient what one could reasonably expect to lose on a proper diet the usual response is four to five pounds per week or more, even from intelligent patients. To lose four pounds in one week would require an intake of 14,000 calories (3,500 calories per pound) less than the body burned, or 2,000 calories per day less than needed. Since few obese patients require as much as 2,000 calories per day total, to lose four pounds per week the patient would have to eat less than nothing—clearly absurd. In fact, a daily intake of 500 calories less than needed is a very satisfactory dietary performance from the long-range point of view. However, this will only lead to a weight loss of one pound weekly ($7 \times 500 = 3,500$).

This analysis bears directly upon the common claim that "I can gain (lose) five to ten pounds overnight." Generally these weight swings follow a large meal. However, most of what is weighed is water, and this is excreted in the urine rather rapidly. In addition, there is solid waste which eventually passes with the feces. Urine, excess extracellular fluid and fecal matter are all within the body, and contribute to total body weight, but are not constituents of body tissues. The temporary retention or excretion of these materials may produce dramatic changes in total body weight, while there is essentially no change in the body tissue weight. Over a longer period of time, e.g. several weeks, shifts in these substances balance out and one can obtain some indication of whether there has been a change in body tissue weight. This assumes that the weight is measured by a reliable scale, at the same time of day, preferably after an elimination and without clothing. Since patients seldom pay attention to these details, and even less often have available a reliable scale, their reports of weight changes are of dubious value.

Unscrupulous diet quacks take advantage of the effects of laxatives and diuretics to convince their clients that they can produce a rapid and dramatic weight loss. Naturally these losses are not sustained, but there is a new crop of victims every day.

The obese patient, constantly searching for magical remedies is always on the alert for the latest fad diet. Since these diets are conceptually and practically unsound, their proponents have lately found themselves either in jail or in litigation. Thus there is a constant need for new fads. Nevertheless, just as surely as nature abhors a vacuum, the demand for fad diets produces a never ending supply —a tribute to the imagination of the hustlers.

Any diet that deviates from a pattern of eating which would be permanently suitable, is *ipso facto* conceptually unsound. Obesity is not a problem for a week or a month, it is a life-long problem. Fad diets actually are harmful since they distract the patient from this essential reality, and only serve to delay his coming to terms with the necessity of learning what and how to eat for the rest of his life. Furthermore, fad diets encourage the natural inclination of the patient to live in the fantasy world of magic, where sooner or later the correct wand will wave away all troubles.

At the risk of redundancy, I shall add that fad diets are not acceptable even to "get the patient started." The problem is not getting started. No matter what method is employed almost all obese patients do well for the first few weeks. It is the need for persistent and consistent dieting that leads to failure.

Finally, in some cases fad diets have actually been shown to be unhealthy, particularly for the obese.

Notions About Disease as a Cause of Obesity

"There must be something physically wrong with me." "It's my glands (endocrines are cited by the more sophisticated)." "It's really mostly fluid, all bloat!" The desire to find some explanation, other than the obvious is exceedingly intense in obese patients.

After all, if they are sick, they are not to blame. Furthermore, it is the doctor's fault because in the first place he does not know enough to find out what is wrong; and secondly, he failed to administer the proper remedy. Emphasis upon miraculous scientific breakthroughs in the lay literature *(most of which, of course, are ultimately shown to have no more value than yesterday's newspaper)*, in conjunction with a multitude of fraudulent publications with promises like "calories don't count," serve to reinforce the notion that there really is some simple medical solution to the obesity problem.

It is particularly popular to blame obesity upon the endocrine system, especially the thyroid gland. In fact, endocrine disease, including hypothyroidism, is never the sole cause of obesity and seldom is even a contributing factor. Nevertheless, it is a rare obese patient who has not been given thyroid hormone at some time in a fruitless attempt at correcting nonexistent hypothyroidism. To add irony to irony, the dosage of thyroid hormone employed is often homeopathic.

The fluid retention problem, upon which obese patients frequently dwell at great length, is an example of a notion about which there is some truth. There is a tendency for fluid retention in obese individuals, especially when dieting. Nevertheless, this fluid ultimately is excreted, whether diuretics are given or not. Fluid retention never contributes more than a fraction of the obese person's superfluous poundage. Fluid retention may be particularly uncomfortable in the week or two preceding menstruation, a time when this problem seems to be annoying even for nonobese women. The use of diuretics may be justifiable to promote fluid excretion, but diuretics do not begin to solve the obesity per se.

Notions About the Role of the Physician

"Why won't you give me some shots or pills to make me lose weight or curb my appetite—if only just to get me started?" "Doctor, you don't want to help me!" Diet pills *(or capsules)* have been consumed by the millions, perhaps by the billions. They come in all sizes, shapes and colors. New models come out yearly like the autos. However, is there any data to suggest that there is less obesity as a result? Should it not be obvious that if any of the many diet medications were truly effective there would be no need for a host of competitors? Although diet pills have been available for many years, where is the study to show that the use of any of these medications has resulted in a significant weight loss in any sizable population of obese patients which was sustained for ten years, or five years, or even two years? There is no convincing evidence that diet pills have made any real contribution to the management of obesity.

On the contrary there are valid objections to the use of these drugs in a weight reduction program, in addition to the potential for abuse. The ordering of drugs serves to reinforce the faulty notion that obesity is the result of some physical abnormality that requires medication to correct. The implication is that weight loss is produced by the pill. Therefore, no weight loss simply means the wrong pills. If the physician attempts to explain the uselessness of diet drugs, unless this is done with great tact and persuasion, it may be interpreted as a rejection of the patient. After all the patient did not come to reduce, but rather to be reduced.

These faulty notions reflect attitudes of the obese patient which constitute a major barrier to the achievement of weight reduction. These attitudes may be summarized as follows:

1. *It is not my fault that I am overweight.*
   a. It is not that I eat too much, it is just that my body does not burn up the food properly.
   b. Furthermore, I have done everything that can be expected of me, including all kinds of diets, diet pills and consultations with many diet specialists.
2. *If anyone is to blame it is the doctor.*
   a. Why doesn't he find out what is wrong with me?
   b. Why doesn't he give me the right medication?
   c. I have paid to be reduced, but have not been helped.
   d. If the greatest minds in medicine are stumped by my problem, what can you expect from me?

Thus, the physician who attempts to treat obesity must deal with a patient quite different from that for which most of his training has prepared him. There are powerful and realistic motivating factors which induce the patient to perpetuate his disease, whereas the cure is unpleasant and protracted. When the patient consults a physician it may not be solely for the purpose of obtaining his advice, for the advice is obvious. The patient may desire and expect magic, and if the physician fails to fulfill these unrealistic expectations, as far as the patient is concerned, the failure is that of the physician, and it is the physician who should bear the onus for the continuing obesity.

Obviously any physician who hopes to accomplish something of lasting value with obese patients cannot play the game by these rules. Therefore establishing proper ground rules should be an item of top priority in any weight reduction regimen. Assisting the patient to understand certain unalterable facts of life will be helpful in this regard.

FACTS OF LIFE FOR THE OBESE

OBESITY RESULTS FROM OVEREATING. This is true for every obese person regardless of age, sex, activity status or the presence of other illness which might affect weight. Overeating does not necessarily imply gluttony. It is possible to eat rather small quantities of food and still be overeating. Overeating simply means eating more than the body needs.

THERE IS NO DISEASE, ENDOCRINE OR OTHERWISE, THE CORRECTION OF WHICH WILL ELIMINATE OBESITY. Patients with hypothyroidism may be obese, but may also be underweight. The average deviation and range of deviation from normal weight is not different from that observed for patients with normal thyroid function. Diabetes mellitus is also associated with obesity. However, it seems more likely that the obesity is an aggravating factor for the diabetes, than that the diabetes causes the obesity. In any event, for both hypothyroidism and diabetes, obesity when present indicates overeating. Neither correction of hypothyroidism nor control of blood sugar will correct the associated obesity without caloric restriction.

ONCE ESTABLISHED, OBESITY IS A PROBLEM FOR LIFE.

THERE IS NO MAGICAL REMEDY FOR OBESITY. There is no magic diet. There are no magic physicians. No physician has any secret remedy not available to all other physicians. No medication ever reduced an obese patient, and no physician ever reduced an obese patient.

THE ONLY WAY TO LOSE WEIGHT IS TO EAT LESS THAN THE BODY NEEDS, CONSISTENTLY. The only way to keep weight down is to continue to curtail food intake for life.

A PROPER MENTAL ATTITUDE IS ESSENTIAL TO WEIGHT REDUCTION. If one thinks of dieting as "starving," "eating nothing," "suffering," "self-denial," "abnormal," it will soon become impossible to persist. The truth is that dieting is eating normally, perhaps for the first time in many years. Dieting restores, preserves and prolongs health and life. Dieting is no more unpleasant than many other experiences which are part of life. Dieting will be less difficult to bear if viewed as a healthier way of living not only for the patient, but for the rest of the family as well.

In addition to hunger in its various forms, many patients develop other symptoms while dieting. These include headache, constipation, weakness, irritability, tension, nervousness and sleeplessness. These symptoms do not mean starvation or serious disease. Concentration on the purposes of the diet and the benefits to be realized will help one tolerate these symptoms. Equally unpleasant and even more severe symptoms can be borne with equanimity by a determined patient. A case in point is the recent popularity of natural childbirth. With proper mental and physical preparation, considerable discomfort can be tolerated without pain medication. The mother chooses to accept this discomfort for the welfare of her baby and other related motivating considerations.

ACCEPTANCE OF THE FACTS OF LIFE IS ESSENTIAL FOR SUCCESSFUL DIETING. If the patient cannot adjust to these realities there is no point in pursuing the matter.

THE PHYSICIAN'S ROLE IN THE TREATMENT OF OBESITY

The treatment of obesity is caloric restriction. I can offer no useful elaboration. I have no special diet, no wonder drug, no new method to foster motivation. In fact, the constructive role of the physician in the management of obesity patients is limited, but may be considered briefly under the following headings:

EVALUATIVE. The physician is needed for the necessary appraisal of emotional, intellectual, and physical resources and limitations upon which decisions as to the suitability of a program of dieting and exercise must be based.

EDUCATIONAL. Instruction in proper eating habits, food selection, and most of all in the elimination of self defeating notions is important for successful treatment.

COUNSELING. Occasionally, the physician may be of assistance in helping the patient make adjustments or accommodations to personal problems at home or work which are aggravating factors. Alternatively, it may be necessary to suggest formal counseling or even psychiatric evaluation.

SUPPORT. The sympathy and understanding of a physician may be helpful, particularly with patients who exhibit strong dependency needs. Reassurance and encouragement by a medical authority can help the patient survive periods of discouragement and depression over lack of progress.

ANALYTICAL. Analysis of diet records for unrecognized sources of "hidden" calories, serial weight, and measurement determinations are useful services which the physician can provide.

AVOID BEING PART OF THE PROBLEM. The physician must avoid assuming an attitude suggesting that by virtue of his special skill and expertise he will solve the patient's problem. Obesity is the patient's problem, and only the patient can solve it. The physician must not allow the patient to manipulate the doctor-patient relationship to place the responsibility for success or failure upon the physician. The physician should not encourage the patient to rely upon drugs or fad diets, but should advise and pursue a long-range perspective of the problem.

THE PHYSICIAN'S REACTION TO THE PERSONALITY OF THE OBESITY PATIENT

The primary purpose of this chapter is to indicate that personality problems with the obesity patient may increase the difficulties of weight reduction. The limited role which the physician may play also has been emphasized. At this point it seems proper to consider the danger that physician attitudes also may serve to perpetuate obesity.

Although it is axiomatic that a physician should not become emotionally involved with his patients, for the obesity patient, adherence to this principle may be difficult. Lacking complete understanding of the underlying pathophysiology, having no specific and effective remedy to offer and appreciating that regardless of what is done, the long-term prospects for control are poor, the physician may feel insecure in his relationship to obesity patients. When an insecure physician faces a hostile patient, the result is hardly conducive to effective problem solving. The physician may completely reject the patient, refusing even to evaluate him on the grounds that it is not a medical problem, and he is too busy taking care of "sick" patients. The rejection may be less overt, but just as complete if the patient is bruskly advised to eat less and exercise by pushing away from the table. Rejection may be compounded by a challenge of veracity if the physician insists that the patient is eating more than is admitted.

In addition to being crude, cruel and ineffective, these approaches signify an abdication of the physician's responsibility to be as helpful as possible, even in a situation for which the prospects do not seem promising. The physician may be able to cope with these patients more effectively if he makes it clear at the outset that he can serve only in an advisory capacity, and that the responsibility for success or failure will remain squarely upon the shoulders of the patient.

PRINCIPLES UNDERLYING A WEIGHT REDUCTION REGIMEN

Dieting

The only way to lose weight is to diet. There are many excellent references available to assist the would-be dieter. Hence it seems necessary to consider the principles or guidelines which must not only be followed, but understood and indeed incorporated as fixed and inflexible habits. I deliberately de-emphasize printed menus or diet lists. One must know how to eat just as he knows how to dress or perform any other routine function in life. Dependency upon written instructions is not only unnecessary, but also an invitation to failure. For what does the dieter do, who is dependent upon the printed word, when faced with the many situations in which it may be impossible or impractical to consult a printed diet? This dieter is simply lost. For reference, and to assist one to expand the variety of a diet, diet books are fine. For the everyday practice of dieting one must use judgment and common sense, based upon a thorough understanding of principles. Therefore, on with the principles:

1. There is no place for sweets on a diet, not occasionally, not for special events, not once a year, not just a taste, none, never. Just as it can become habitual to desire sweets, it can become habitual to avoid them. Only total abstinence can promote the development of this habit.

2. Pure starch foods also should be eliminated. This includes bread, potatoes, noodles, rice, spaghetti, crackers, corn and the like in all of the various forms in which they may appear. These foods serve no essential function other than to increase obesity. On the surface this may seem a rather harsh rule, but again I would emphasize that once it has become habitual to avoid these foods, it will then seem as unnatural to eat them as now it may seem essential.

3. Fatty and fried foods should be avoided. This includes gravy, the skin of poultry, pork, duck, goose, prime beef (use choice instead) and salad dressing (other than the low calorie varieties). Choose white meat over dark in poultry. Bake, boil and broil. Use greaseless pans for frying. Trim off all fat. Fish is a particularly good source of protein. Avoid tuna or salmon packed in oil; use the water packed variety.

4. Do eat green vegetables, cooked or raw. Avoid yellow vegetables—e.g. corn, carrots, squash, and also legumes (peas and beans).

5. In the dairy category take no cream, use skim milk. Cottage cheese is good, especially with salad; brick cheese in small quantities is acceptable.

6. Fruits are necessary, but in limited quantities. Orange, grapefruit, cantaloupe, apple, pear, banana, peach, plum; but avoid grapes, cherries, watermelon and dried fruits, especially raisins. Fruits should be limited to one selection daily.

7. Alcoholic beverages are absolutely prohibited. They are not nutritious, yet are high in calories.

8. Soft drinks, other than the low calorie type are absolutely prohibited.

9. Low calorie prepared foods for dieters, such as canned fruits, salad dressings and many others are helpful to add variety. However, avoid low calorie bread, cookies or other starch-like substances. They only encourage the desire for the real thing, exactly contrary to our wish to develop the habit of avoiding these foods. Furthermore, they are not truly low in calories.

10. Food should be distributed in three meals. Snacking is prohibited other than celery. Note: Carrot sticks are not low in calories.

11. The size of portions should be estimated and the adequacy of the estimate determined by the course of monthly weights. If the weight is dropping at the rate of ½ to 1½ pounds per week, fine;

if not, cut the size of portions until success is achieved.

12. Initially all food eaten should be recorded. Analysis of these records may be helpful if progress is not satisfactory.

These are the key dietary principles by which the person with a weight problem must live. Before leaving the discussion of diet, it will be useful to consider how one should handle certain special situations which must be faced with equanimity if one is to be comfortable with dieting.

1. What should the dieter do when invited to a friend's home for dinner?
   a. Plan ahead. Know what types of food you are going to eat and what you are going to say if someone thinks you are not eating enough. If you are not prepared you will be vulnerable to attack by thoughtless and boorish people.
   b. Do not say you are dieting under any circumstances. This will expose you to ridicule and embarrassment.
   c. Take some of everything that is offered, but don't eat anything you shouldn't, and no more than you should of what you can eat. Your hostess wants you to take food, she really doesn't care, and likely will not notice whether you eat it.
   d. If you are faced with a particularly crude hostess or fellow guest who presses you to eat or drink that which you know you must avoid, simply inform the party that you have tasted it and it is delicious, but you cannot take any more (or any at all, in the case of alcohol) because you are having some special tests at your doctor's office tomorrow, and you are limited in what you can eat. Emphasize how expensive the tests are, and it wouldn't do to spoil them. This answer will drive off the most insistent of boors, and permit you to enjoy socializing without ruining your diet.

2. What about dining out on that special occasion?
   a. Again, plan ahead.
   b. Order an appetizer, e.g., fruit, seafood with lemon, but not cocktail sauce.
   c. Order a salad with lemon and salt—do not ask for low calorie dressing, to avoid embarrassment and calling attention to the fact that you are dieting.
   d. Order a green vegetable.

e. Nibble on the celery.

f. Order fish or a small steak as your main course.

g. Finish with coffee and you have had enough to eat.

Exercise

Exercise is an important supplement to dieting in any weight reduction program. Everyone can exercise; some can do it more vigorously than others; all who have not done it on a regular basis will have to build up tolerance gradually. Overdoing too soon can be very dangerous, particularly for the obese. Before beginning on an exercise program one should have a thorough physical examination, including a stress test of some sort to check on the cardiac status.

Exercise includes everything from simple repetitive movement of the limbs by a bedridden patient to the more vigorous competitive sports. The same principles apply:

1. Exercise must be daily.

2. Exercise must be for some duration, preferably an hour at a time, or total during the day.

3. The best exercise is the exercise which is fun, for that is the only exercise which will be pursued for life. Tennis, squash, handball, and racket ball are some of the best exercises because they offer the challenge of competition. Swimming, jogging, and bike riding are fine. Calisthenics of one sort or another may prove to be too much of a discipline for most people to continue indefinitely.

4. One should start off slowly and build up the tolerance over six months or more depending upon his physical condition.

Exercise can take many forms other than formal sports. For example, one should always park as far from the entrance to work as possible, and jog from the car to the door. If you work in a high rise building, get off three floors short of yours and walk up; walk down five or six flights. Never ride when walking is reasonable. Do your own yard work, painting, snow shoveling. Analyze your daily activities looking for every way possible to increase your energy consumption in routine activities.

Weighing

The dieter should avoid weighing more than once monthly. The average successful dieter will lose ½ to 1½ pounds weekly. This is too small an amount to measure accurately on the usual home scale, particularly if one realizes that fluid changes may easily exceed this amount. Only larger sustained weight changes are significant. There is nothing more discouraging than dieting for several days and seeing no results on the scale. Worse yet, is the observation of a "loss" of two or three pounds overnight, only to "gain" it back the next day. Remember, if you take care of the diet, the weight will take care of itself.

Group Therapy

There are a number of lay organizations which offer group situations in which dieters can share their experiences and attempt to motivate one another. In some instances they advocate dieting concepts which may not be appropriate, or set unrealistic goals. Nevertheless, I believe these groups may be helpful for some people and I do not discourage participation.

Psychotherapy

For some people obesity, and the inability to correct it by dietary measurements, is a manifestation of a more profound emotional disturbance. Perhaps every unsuccessful dieter should consider a psychiatric evaluation, particularly if he has the insight to appreciate that he is unable to cooperate consistently with the weight reduction regimen. Unfortunately, this recommendation may not lead to success in all instances. Psychiatric counseling is beyond the means of many people. Not all psychiatrists are able to deal efficiently with the problem of obesity. The life-long nature of the problem presents a limiting factor upon what may be achieved with psychiatric help.

Conclusions

1. There is no magic road to weight reduction. No one can reduce the obese patient except the patient.

2. Success on a weight reduction regimen demands an all out dedication to a comprehensive effort at changing ones life style so that reduction in caloric intake and increased caloric consumption (increased activity) become as natural and habitual as sleeping and breathing.

3. Planning ahead is essential to avoid the abundance of social traps which lie in wait for the unwary dieter.

4. The task is long and hard, the temptations are many, even though success may be long delayed, one should not give up, for the rewards at last are great—both physical and mental.

GLOSSARY OF TERMS AND PHRASES USEFUL IN UNDERSTANDING THE FUNCTION AND DISEASES OF THE THYROID GLAND

Antibiotic

A medication to kill germs employed in the treatment of infection.

Antithyroid Drugs

Medications which curtail the ability of the thyroid gland to produce thyroid hormone (e.g. propylthiouracil or methimazole). These medications may be useful in the treatment of hyperthyroidism.

Autonomous Function

Function which persists without regard to any regulating factors which arise outside the functioning tissue itself; independent function. Some thyroid nodules function autonomously.

Autonomously Functioning Thyroid Nodule

A nodule of thyroid tissue which functions independently of the normal pituitary-thyroid feedback autoregulatory mechanism.

BEI

Butanol-extractable iodine. A crude method of measuring blood levels of thyroxine. This test has been rendered obsolete by more specific and reliable techniques.

BMR

Basal metabolic rate. One of the first tests of thyroid function. The test measures oxygen consumption. It is now considered too unreliable for accurate diagnosis in thyroid disease.

Colloid

The gelatinous material which fills the follicles of the thyroid gland and contains stored thyroid hormone.

Cretin

The end result of severe hypothyroidism present from birth or infancy. The patient is mentally retarded, stunted in growth, and has the other characteristic findings of hypothyroidism. Goiter may be a prominent feature of the disease if the basis of the thyroid hormone deficiency is inefficient hormonal synthesis. There will be no goiter if, as a result of an accident of heredity, thyroid tissue is absent.

Degeneration

A process whereby body organs and tissues undergo a progressive deterioration in vitality and functional capacity. This is frequently seen as part of the wear and tear of aging or overwork, or both.

Desiccated Thyroid

The first commercially available form of thyroid hormone. This product is a crude preparation of animal thyroid gland material, may prove unreliable in dosage, and may not be well absorbed from the gastrointestinal tract.

Disease

A general term referring to any abnormality of the body or its parts from the most minor to the most serious.

Enzymes

Chemical substances which are important in many of the processes whereby materials necessary for body function are produced. For example, the synthesis of thyroid hormone requires a number of steps, each of which is controlled by a specific enzyme.

Esophagus

The tubular structure through which food passes from the throat to the stomach.

Euthyroid State

The condition in which there is a normal amount of thyroid

hormone available to the body. (See *Hyperthyroidism* and *Hypothyroidism*).

Exophthalmic Goiter

A form of hyperthyroidism in which there is hyperfunction of the entire gland, associated with protrusion of the eyes (*exophthalmos*).

Feedback Autoregulartory System

Feedback autoregulation of function is a special property of endocrine glands. The pituitary gland (or master gland) produces stimulating hormones which activate other endocrine glands (target or subordinate glands) causing them to secrete their products into the blood. Rising blood levels of these hormones in turn are fed back to a sampling center at the base of the brain, close to the pituitary, and the pituitary secretion of stimulating hormone is turned off. In the pituitary-thyroid autoregulation, low blood levels of thyroid hormone lead to pituitary secretion of thyroid stimulating hormone (TSH) which travels through the blood to the thyroid gland increasing the secretion of thyroid hormone. As blood levels of thyroid hormone rise the change is detected at the brain, and pituitary TSH secretion decreases. When thyroid blood levels fall, TSH is once again released in increased quantities to activate the thyroid gland.

Follicle

One of the many hollow spherical structures of which the thyroid gland is composed. The follicles are lined by the active thyroid gland cells which produce thyroid hormone. This hormone is then stored in the colloid contained within the cavities of the follicles until needed.

Free Thyroxine Index (FTI)

An estimate of the active (unbound) form of thyroxine in the blood. See Chapter 3.

Gland, Endocrine

Glands are body organs which have the function of producing some necessary substance. The endocrine glands are special in that they release their products (hormones) directly into the blood.

Goiter

Any enlargement of the thyroid gland is called a goiter. If the enlargement is generalized the goiter is called diffuse, if localized into one or more lumps it is called nodular. The terms "inward" and "outward" goiter are *not* medical terms and have no significant meaning.

Graves' Disease

A form of hyperthyroidism associated with diffuse goiter and exophthalmos described by a British physician, Robert J. Graves. (See *Exophthalmic Goiter*.)

Hashimoto's Disease

A form of chronic inflammation of thyroid, often associated with goiter and hypothyroidism, described by a Japanese physician, by whose name the disease is known.

Hormone

A chemical substance produced by an endocrine gland, secreted into the blood stream to produce its effects at one or more locations remote from its gland of origin. Thyroid hormone is the hormone produced by the thyroid gland. Other familiar hormones include cortisol from the adrenal gland, estrogen from the ovary, and testosterone from the testis.

Hyperthyroidism

The disorder which results from an excess of thyroid hormone within the body. This excess thyroid hormone usually comes from an abnormal thyroid gland, but may result from overdosage of medication containing thyroid hormone.

Hypothyroidism

The disorder which results from an inadequate quantity of thyroid hormone available to the body.

Iodine

An essential element in the production of thyroid hormone.

Isotope, Radioactive

An unstable form of an element which has the property of giving off radioactivity. Radioactive isotopes (more recently the term "nuclide" is preferred) are by-products of the nuclear reactor and are useful in medicine for both diagnostic testing and treatment.

Larynx

A muscular cartilaginous structure in the middle of the neck which contains the vocal cords, and by means of which the voice is produced.

Methimazole

A medication used to reduce the function of the thyroid gland in hyperthyroidism. The trade name *Tapazole*® is more commonly used.

Myxedema

This term is usually used to imply a severe degree of hypothyroidism (See Fig. 1 Chap. 6). Some physicians use the word interchangeably with "hypothyroidism," and make no distinction as to the severity of the disorder.

Neoplasm

A growth, made up of abnormal tissue which may be either benign or malignant.

Nodular Goiter

This term is applied to a thyroid gland which may or may not be diffusely enlarged, but has one or more distinct nodules (see *Nodule*).

Nodule

A small lump, usually between the size of a pea and that of a golf ball.

Objective Data

The results of evaluation or testing which is entirely independent of the patient's thoughts and opinions, e.g. a blood count, or the findings of a physician's physical examination (see *Subjective Data*).

Palpitation

A sensation of forceful, irregular, or rapid heart beat. Normally, one is unaware of the beating of the heart. In hyperthyroidism, or with certain heart disorders the complaint of palpitation may be quite distressing.

Parathyroid Glands

These are tiny glands, usually four in number, which are located adjacent to the thyroid gland. They produce a hormone which controls the level of calcium in the blood. The prefix "para" means *near to*. Since these glands are adjacent to the thyroid, they were named parathyroid glands long before their function was understood. Because of their nearness to the thyroid gland and their small size, during thyroid surgery they can easily be inadvertently removed, or so damaged that function is impaired.

PBI

Protein-bound iodine. An early, now obsolescent, test by which one can estimate thyroid hormone blood levels.

Pituitary Gland

The pituitary gland (or master gland) is a small gland, about the size of an olive, which lies in a special bony compartment in the base of the skull. There are connections with a portion of the brain called the hypothalamus. Within the hypothalamus are sensitive detection centers which constantly measure levels of various hormones in the blood and send information to the pituitary which stimulates function of target glands (thyroid, adrenal, ovary, testis) (See *Feedback Autoregulatory System*).

Pretibial Myxedema

A painless thickening and darkening of the skin over the lower outer portion of the leg. This is a confusing term, because we have already associated the word "myxedema" with hypothyroidism (See *Myxedema*). Yet, pretibial myxedema is a change in the skin of the lower leg seen only in Graves' disease.

Prognosis

An estimate as to the probable course, and outcome of an illness.

Radioimmunoassay (RIA)

A new method for measuring substances in the blood which

are present in very low concentrations. See Chapter 3.

T_3(RIA): A measurement of the blood levels of T_3 by the RIA method.

TSH(RIA): A measurement of the blood level of TSH by the RIA method.

RAI

Radioactive iodine, ^{131}I, the principal radioactive isotope of naturally occurring iodine which is used for diagnostic and therapeutic purposes in medicine.

RAI Uptake

A test of thyroid function in which the take-up of RAI by the thyroid gland in a given period of time (usually twenty-four hours) is measured.

Scan

A recording in picture form of the distribution of RAI uptake within the thyroid gland. The picture is produced by a machine called a scanner.

Secretion

The process whereby a gland releases its product (into the blood in the case of endocrine glands).

Suppression Test

A test of the integrity of the pituitary-thyroid feedback autoregulatory system. Normally the administration of thyroid hormone suppresses pituitary TSH release, and this suppression can be shown by a fall in the RAI uptake. In hyperthyroidism, autoregulation is deranged, and the RAI uptake is not suppressible.

Subjective Data

Information supplied by the patient which cannot be confirmed by the physician's observation or laboratory testing. For example, a description of the quality, severity, and location of a pain. (See *Objective Data*).

Tapazole®

Trade name for methimazole. A commonly enmployed medication to reduce the function of the thyroid gland in hyperthyroid conditions.

Thymus Gland

A gland-like structure located in the upper front part of the chest. It is largest in infancy and childhood, and becomes smaller spontaneously with age. Its function is not fully understood, but appears to relate to body defense mechanisms. In the past, an enlarged thymus in an infant was feared as a possible cause of strangulation. Many infants were treated with x-ray. A significant proportion of these patients developed thyroid cancer ten or more years later.

Thyroiditis, Chronic: (Hashimoto's Disease)

A chronic inflammatory disorder of the thyroid gland, of unknown cause, which leads to the development of a very firm goiter and usually some degree of hypothyroidism.

Thyroiditis, Subacute

An inflammation of the thyroid gland which seems to be caused by one of several types of viruses, and causes pain and swelling of the thyroid. The process usually subsides spontaneously, but medication may be required for relief.

Thyroxine (T_4)

This is the principal hormone secreted by the thyroid gland. The abbreviation T_4 stems from the fact that each molecule has four atoms of iodine. T_4 is available for oral administration under the trade names *Synthroid®* and *Letter.®* See also *Triiodothyronine (T_3)*.

$T_4(D)$

A new method for measuring the blood level of thyroxine specifically.

Toxic

This term means hyperthyroid. It is often used preceding the type of goiter as in toxic diffuse goiter.

Toxic Autonomously Functioning Nodule

A solitary overactive thyroid nodule producing hyperthyroidism. See Chapter 5.

Toxic Goiter, Diffuse

A synonym for Graves' disease.

Toxic Goiter, Nodular

Similar to toxic diffuse goiter, but rather than a smooth generalized enlargement, the goiter contains one or more nodules. Management may be somewhat different as a result.

Trachea

The windpipe

Triiodothyronine (T₃)

The second hormone produced by the thyroid gland. Each molecule has only three atoms of iodine, compared to four for T_4. This reduction in iodine content is accompanied by about a fourfold increase in potency. See also *Thyroxine (T₄)*.

TSH

Thyroid-stimulating hormone, a product of the pituitary gland which stimulates thyroid gland function.

Tumor

Any swelling or mass of tissue whether benign or malignant. The word "tumor" is generally applied to larger lumps than those called nodules, but there is overlap in the use of these two words.

Ultrasound

A new diagnostic test to differentiate cystic from solid thyroid nodules. See Chapters 3 and 7.

INDEX

111